OSCE Guide for the ABA Applied Examination

OSCE Guide for the ABA Applied Examination

Milo Engoren
Professor
Department of Anesthesiology, University of Michigan, USA

Sean Neill
Assistant Professor
Department of Anesthesiology, Pharmacology & Therapeutics
University of British Columbia, Canada

William Simpson
Consultant, Department of Cardiothoracic Anaesthesia, Lancashire Cardiac Centre, UK

Andrew Davies
Consultant in Cardiothoracic Anaesthesia and Critical Care, University Hospital of South Manchester NHS Foundation Trust, UK

Peter Frank
Consultant in Anaesthesia and Intensive Care Medicine, Lancashire Teaching Hospitals NHS Foundation Trust, UK

Simon Maguire
Consultant in Anaesthesia, University Hospital of South Manchester NHS Foundation Trust, UK

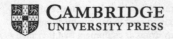
CAMBRIDGE
UNIVERSITY PRESS

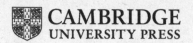
CAMBRIDGE
UNIVERSITY PRESS

Shaftesbury Road, Cambridge CB2 8EA, United Kingdom

One Liberty Plaza, 20th Floor, New York, NY 10006, USA

477 Williamstown Road, Port Melbourne, VIC 3207, Australia

314–321, 3rd Floor, Plot 3, Splendor Forum, Jasola District Centre, New Delhi – 110025, India

103 Penang Road, #05–06/07, Visioncrest Commercial, Singapore 238467

Cambridge University Press is part of Cambridge University Press & Assessment, a department of the University of Cambridge.

We share the University's mission to contribute to society through the pursuit of education, learning and research at the highest international levels of excellence.

www.cambridge.org
Information on this title: www.cambridge.org/9781107594999

DOI: 10.1017/9781316476864

First published 2017

A catalogue record for this publication is available from the British Library

Library of Congress Cataloging-in-Publication data
Names: Engoren, Milo, author. | Neill, Sean. | Simpson, William.
Title: OSCE guide for the ABA applied examination / Milo Engoren, Professor, Department of Anesthesiology, University of Michigan, USA, Sean Neill and William Simpson.
Description: Cambridge, United Kingdom ; New York, NY : Cambridge University Press, 2017. | Includes bibliographical references and index.
Identifiers: LCCN 2017022456 | ISBN 9781107594999 (paperback)
Subjects: LCSH: Anesthesiology – Examinations, questions, etc.
Classification: LCC RD82.3 .E54 2017 | DDC 617.9/6–dc23
LC record available at https://lccn.loc.gov/2017022456

ISBN   978-1-107-59499-9   Paperback

....

Contents

Section 8. Resuscitation and Simulation

Section 9. Procedures

Section 10. Monitoring and Measurement

Preface

The Objective Structured Clinical Examination (OSCE) is designed to measure if the examinee can do things. Using written and oral examinations, the examinees have already shown that they know things, have sufficient knowledge to be anesthesiologists, but are they just "book smart?" When I started in medical school, certifying examinations were mostly written but some had an oral component where examinees needed to show that they could think and act like a consultant. Critics complained that these examinations did not show how the examinee would perform in a real situation. Some specialties and programs, mostly outside the United States, developed clinical examinations using real patients. Typically, the examinees would rotate amongst several patients and they would either be observed or, more usually, questioned afterwards to measure what history they had elicited and what physical findings they had noticed. These examinations suffered from the variability in the patients. While real, some patients gave better histories, some had better (easier) physical examinations. (Palpating splenomegaly in an obese patient is challenging.) They also suffered from the unstructured questions the examiners used on the examinees. Different examiners asked different questions with a different degree of thoroughness.

When I was a resident, I was an examiner for a physician assistants' physical examination test. Students came in, I read with them the clinical scenario, and they performed a focused physical examination. I had a checklist and for each item on the list that they did, I checked it off. They could do superfluous items. There was no credit for these, but also no penalty. The total number of correctly performed items translated into a score and a pass or fail. I wondered why physician assistants but not physicians needed to show clinical competence. Over the succeeding years, I have worked with a few physicians who were very smart, had top scores on all the written examinations. They could cite the 20 most common causes of chest pain, but didn't know what to do when faced with a real patient with chest pain.

In the succeeding decades, the calls for an examination that tests clinical skills have increased. Fortunately, the science of the OSCE has advanced. Tests are carefully constructed for validity. Examiners are trained. Clinical patients are trained. This minimizes other variability as much as possible, leaving the examinee as the major source of variation in performance. Patients will give the same answers to the same questions – if asked by the examinee.

During medical school and residency, few students and residents get many (or any) opportunities to do and practice the OSCE. Much as auscultating a chest or reading an X-ray, practice builds skills. We offer this book as a helpful guide to you to build your OSCE skills. It presents a number of clinical scenarios and shows how to approach each one.

Acknowledgements

Many thanks to Dr. Andreas Erdmann for permitting the reproduction of the anatomy images taken from his *Concise Anatomy for Anaesthesia*. Without his help and support, the task of constructing the anatomy section would have been almost impossible. We would also like to thank Dr. James Howard, Radiology Registrar, North Western Deanery, for his help with the X-ray films and Dr. James Mitchell, Cardiology Registrar, North Western Deanery, for his help with the ECGs. We would also like to extend our sincerest thanks to the Cambridge University Press and Dr. William Simpson for allowing us to reuse the images from the *Primary FRCA: OSCEs in Anaesthesia* book.

1 Trachea

Candidate's Instructions

Look at this cross-section taken at the level of C5. Answer the following questions.

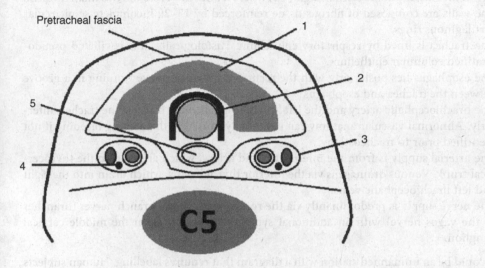

Pretracheal fascia

1
2
3
4
5

C5

Questions

1. Label the structures 1–5.
2. What are the proximal and distal borders of the trachea?
3. What forms the wall of the trachea?
4. Which type of mucosa lines the trachea?
5. What lies immediately posterior to the trachea?
6. Which major vascular structures traverse the trachea anteriorly?
7. What is the blood supply to the trachea?
8. What is the nerve supply of the trachea?

Answers

1. 1. Thyroid gland
   2. Thyroid cartilage
   3. Carotid sheath
   4. Vagus nerve
   5. Esophagus

2. The trachea begins proximally at the lower border of the cricoid cartilage (C6) and terminates distally at the sternal angle (T4) where it bifurcates into the two main bronchi.

3. The walls are composed of fibrous tissue reinforced by 15–20 incomplete semicircular cartilaginous rings.

4. The trachea is lined by respiratory epithelium. Histologically, this is ciliated pseudo-stratified columnar epithelium.

5. The esophagus lies posteriorly with the recurrent laryngeal nerve running in a groove between the trachea and esophagus.

6. The brachiocephalic artery and the left brachiocephalic vein traverse the trachea anteriorly. Abnormal vascular anatomy can potentially cause life-threatening bleeding if not identified prior to tracheostomy.

7. The arterial supply is from the inferior thyroid artery, which arises from the thyrocervical trunk. Venous drainage is via the inferior thyroid veins, which drain into the right and left brachiocephalic veins.

8. The nerve supply is predominantly via the recurrent laryngeal branch nerves (branches of the vagus nerve) with an additional sympathetic supply from the middle cervical ganglion.

This could be an unmanned station with a diagram that requires labelling. Human subjects may be used; therefore, you should be able to recognize anatomical landmarks and explain the path of nerves, blood vessels and muscles and their relations to the trachea.

2 Brachial Plexus

Candidate's Instructions

The following is a diagram of the brachial plexus. Please follow the instructions and answer the questions carefully.

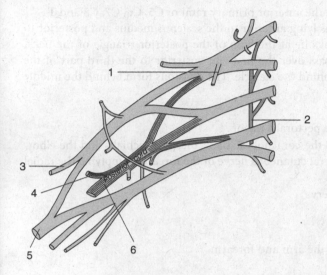

Adapted from Gray H. *Gray's Anatomy*. 1918. Image in the public domain.

Questions

1. Label the structures 1–6.
2. What are the origins of the brachial plexus?
3. Describe the course of the brachial plexus until it reaches the clavicle.
4. What are the branches of the lateral cord?
5. What are the branches of the medial cord?
6. How would you perform a block of the plexus using an axillary approach?
7. Which nerves may be missed using the axillary approach?
8. What complications are associated with supraclavicular nerve blocks?

Answers

1. 1. Nerve to subclavius
   2. Long thoracic nerve
   3. Musculocutaneous nerve
   4. Axillary nerve
   5. Median nerve
   6. Radial nerve

2. The brachial plexus arises from the anterior primary rami of C5, C6, C7, C8 and T1.

3. The plexus emerges as five roots lying anterior to the scalenus medius and posterior to the scalenus anterior. The trunks lie at the base of the posterior triangle of the neck, where they are palpable, and pass over the first rib, posterior to the third part of the subclavian artery, to descend behind the clavicle. The divisions form behind the middle third of the clavicle.

4. Branches of the lateral cord:
   - Lateral pectoral nerve to the pectoralis major
   - Musculocutaneous nerve to the corachobrachialis, biceps, brachialis and the elbow joint. It continues as the lateral cutaneous nerve of the forearm, supplying the radial surface of the forearm
   - Lateral part of the medial nerve

5. Branches of the medial cord:
   - Medial pectoral nerve
   - Medial cutaneous nerves of the arm and forearm
   - Ulnar nerve
   - Medial part of median nerve

6. Perform a PDEQ check:
   - *Patient*: procedure explained, full consent obtained, intravenous access, supine with a pillow under the head, arm abducted with elbow flexed and shoulder rotated so that the hand lies next to the head on the pillow
   - *Drugs*: local anesthetic (skin and injectate); full resuscitation drugs should be available
   - *Equipment*: nerve stimulator and 50-mm insulated nerve stimulator needle. Full monitoring as per ASA guidelines

   Note: ultrasound-guided regional blocks are becoming more popular due to improved efficacy and safety profiles; opt for ultrasound if you have been trained to use it.

   - Position the patient appropriately and identify the axillary artery. Draw a line down from the anterior axillary fold (insertion of pectoralis major) crossing the artery
   - After cleaning and draping the skin, infiltrate local anesthetic subcutaneously
   - Fix the artery between your index and middle finger and insert a needle to pass above or below the artery
   - Pass the needle 45 degrees to the skin, angled proximally to a depth of 10–15 mm, aiming either above the artery (median, musculocutaneous nerves), below the artery (ulnar nerve) or below and behind the artery (radial nerve)

- If using a nerve stimulator, adequate proximity to each nerve is indicated by motor responses produced at 0.2–0.4 mA
- If using ultrasound, the proximity of the needle to the correct nerve can be clearly visualized. Most anesthesiologists would use an in-plane approach for this purpose
- After negative aspiration at 5 mL increments, inject 15 to 25 mL of levobupivicaine, ropivicaine or lidocaine, depending on your desired onset and duration of the block
- Do not inject if blood is aspirated or resistance is felt on injection

7. The axillary approach may miss the intercostobrachial nerve supplying the superomedial surface of the arm and the musculocutaneous nerve. The intercostobrachial nerve can be blocked by subcutaneous infiltration.

8. Complications include:
- Intravascular injection of local anesthetic
- Temporary and permanent nerve damage
- Bleeding
- Failure
- Phrenic nerve palsy
- Recurrent laryngeal nerve palsy
- Pneumothorax

Brachial plexus anatomy may be tested by asking how you would perform a brachial plexus block on a human subject or mannequin. Being able to draw a schematic diagram of the plexus in 10 seconds will not help if the question asks about the anatomical relationships of the plexus in the neck. Detailed knowledge of the neck and upper limb anatomy is vital for safe anesthetic practice.

3 Great Veins of the Neck

Candidate's Instructions

Look at the given diagram and answer the following questions.

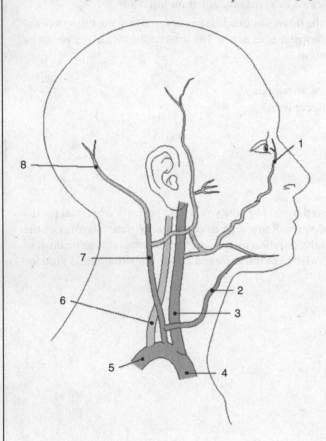

Erdmann A. *Concise Anatomy for Anaesthesia*. Cambridge. 2007. Reproduced with permission.

Questions

1. Label the structures 1–8.
2. Which sinuses combine to form the internal jugular vein?
3. What is the relationship between the internal jugular vein and the carotid artery?
4. Where does the internal jugular vein terminate?
5. Which veins combine to form the external jugular vein?
6. Where do the anterior and external jugular veins join?

Answers

1. 1. Facial vein
   2. Anterior jugular vein
   3. Right internal jugular vein
   4. Right brachiocephalic (innominate) vein
   5. Right subclavian vein
   6. Right vertebral vein
   7. External jugular vein
   8. Posterior auricular vein

2. The sigmoid sinuses and inferior petrosal sinuses combine to form the internal jugular vein, which then passes through the jugular foramen at the base of the skull.

3. The internal jugular vein lies posterior to the carotid artery at the level of C2, postero-lateral at C3, and then lateral to the artery at C4. The vein and artery are contained within the carotid sheath along with the vagus nerve.

4. The internal jugular vein terminates behind the sternoclavicular joint as it unites with the subclavian vein to form the brachiocephalic vein.

5. The external jugular vein arises from the junction of the posterior auricular vein and the posterior division of the retromandibular vein. It lies within the superficial tissues of the neck.

6. The external and anterior jugular veins pierce the deep fascia of the neck, usually posterior to the clavicular head of sternocleidomastoid, and unite before draining into the subclavian vein behind the midpoint of the clavicle.

This station is unlikely to involve demonstrating the anatomy on a human subject. It may touch on central venous cannulation but this is commonly asked in a separate station.

4 Antecubital Fossa

Candidate's Instructions

Look at the given model and answer the questions that follow.

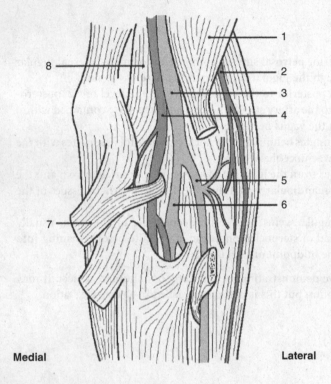

Erdmann A. *Concise Anatomy for Anaesthesia*. Cambridge. 2007. Reproduced with permission.

Questions

1. Label the structures 1–8.
2. What are the borders of the antecubital fossa?
3. What are the contents of the antecubital fossa?
4. What is the path of the radial nerve through the antecubital fossa?
5. Where does the ulnar nerve traverse the elbow joint?
6. How would you block the median nerve at the elbow?

Answers

1. 1. Biceps
   2. Radial nerve
   3. Brachial artery
   4. Median nerve
   5. Radial artery
   6. Ulnar artery
   7. Pronator teres
   8. Brachialis

2. The borders are as follows:

Proximally	– a line between the humeral epicondyles
Laterally	– brachioradialis
Medially	– pronator teres
The floor	– supinator and brachialis
The roof	– deep fascia with median cubital vein and median cutaneous nerve on top

3. The antecubital fossa contains the median, radial and posterior interosseous nerves, the brachial artery (dividing into radial and ulnar arteries) and the biceps tendon.

4. The radial nerve descends in the upper arm, lying between the medial and long heads of the triceps, and enters the antecubital fossa between the lateral epicondyle of the humerus and the musculospiral groove. It runs just laterally to the biceps tendon and under the brachioradialis before dividing into its superficial and deep branches.

5. The ulnar nerve arises medially to the axillary artery and continues medially to the brachial artery, lying on the corachobrachialis, to the midpoint of the humerus. Here it leaves the anterior compartment by passing posteriorly through the medial intermuscular septum with the superior ulnar collateral artery. It lies between the intermuscular septum and the medial head of triceps, passing posteriorly to the medial humeral epicondyle, and enters the forearm between the two heads of flexor carpi ulnaris.

6. Once you have explained the procedure to the patient and have prepared your drugs and equipment:
   - Flex the elbow and mark the elbow crease
   - Identify the brachial artery on this line and mark a point just medial to the artery
   - Clean and drape the area and use a fully aseptic technique
   - Direct your insulated stimulator needle 45 degrees to the skin, aiming proximally
   - At 10–15 mm, a pop or click will be felt (bicipital aponeurosis)
   - Electrical stimulation with 0.2–0.4 mA should elicit finger flexion (pronation alone is inadequate)
   - After negative aspiration, slowly inject 5 mL of your chosen local anesthetic solution to block the nerve

Again note that modern anesthetic practice may well employ the use of ultrasound for a median nerve block. If you have been trained in its use and are happy with the technique, then use that approach.

5 Ankle Block

Candidate's Instructions

In this station you will be asked questions regarding the anatomy of the ankle.

(a)

(b)

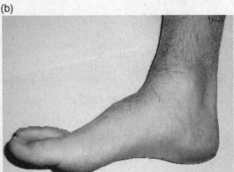

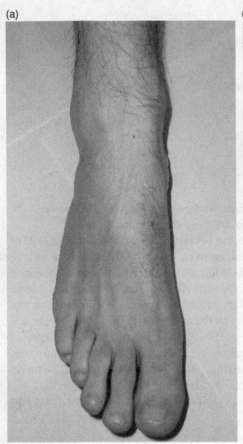

Questions

1. What nerves are you targeting when performing an ankle block?
2. From which spinal nerves does each of these nerves originate?
3. Show me on this volunteer where you would block said nerves?
4. Briefly describe how to block the deep peroneal nerve.
5. What are the indications for an ankle block?
6. What local anesthetic mixtures can you use?
7. What dose of epinephrine would you use to prolong the block?

Answers

1. A successful ankle block needs to target four cutaneous branches of the sciatic nerve: posterior tibial nerve, sural nerve, deep peroneal nerve and superficial peroneal nerve. In addition, target one cutaneous branch of the femoral nerve: saphenous nerve.

2. The origins of these nerves are given as follows:

Posterior tibial	L5–S3
Sural	L5–S2
Deep peroneal	L4–S2
Superficial peroneal	L4–S2
Saphenous	L3–L4

3.

(c)

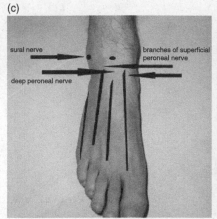

(d)

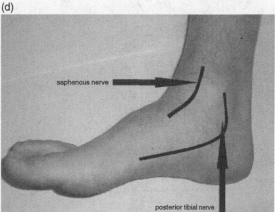

4. This is only a brief question so there is little time for a full procedural explanation:
   - Discuss the risks and benefits of the procedure with the patient and obtain consent
   - Ensure you have full monitoring equipment and a trained assistant
   - Assemble your equipment, clean the area and drape appropriately
   - Don sterile gloves, hat and mask
   - Feel for the groove just lateral to the tendon of the extensor hallucis longus
   - Insert the needle perpendicular to the skin until bone is felt, withdraw slightly and after a negative aspiration, inject 2–4 mL of local anesthetic
   - You may choose a "fan technique" or ask to use ultrasound if you so wish

5. Ankle blocks can be used for any foot and toe surgery.

6. Suitable local anesthetics include 2% lidocaine, 0.5% bupivacaine and 0.5% ropivacaine. Obviously, speed of onset and the duration of the block are dictated by your choice of local anesthetic.

7. **None!** This is a trick question. Using epinephrine for an ankle block is ill advised due to the potential for peripheral ischemia (also the case for hand blocks).

This station lends itself to demonstration of an ankle block on a volunteer and is likely to concentrate on the course and distribution of the nerves involved.

6 Circle of Willis

Candidate's Instructions

Look at the given diagram and answer the following questions.

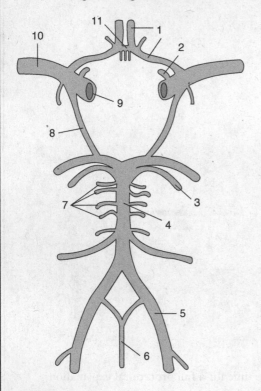

Adapted from Gray H. *Gray's Anatomy*. 1918. Image in the public domain.

Questions

1. Label the structures 1–11.
2. Which arteries supply the Circle of Willis?
3. Where do they enter the skull?
4. What is normal cerebral blood flow?
5. How does the blood flow to white matter and grey matter differ?
6. List the factors affecting cerebral blood flow.
7. Describe the production and circulation of the cerebrospinal fluid (CSF).

Answers

1. 1. Anterior cerebral artery
    2. Ophthalmic artery
    3. Superior cerebellar artery
    4. Basilar artery
    5. Vertebral artery
    6. Anterior spinal artery
    7. Pontine arteries
    8. Posterior communicating artery
    9. Internal carotid artery
    10. Middle cerebral artery
    11. Anterior communicating artery

2. The Circle of Willis is formed from both internal carotid arteries and both vertebral arteries (which form the basilar artery).

3. The internal carotid arteries enter via the carotid canal while the vertebral arteries enter through the foramen magnum.

4. Normal cerebral blood flow is around 15% of the cardiac output = 750 mL/min. This equates to roughly 50 mL/100 g/min.

5. Grey matter receives a higher proportion of blood flow than white matter, 70 mL/100 g/min versus 20 mL/100 g/min, respectively.

6. The factors influencing cerebral blood flow are legion and include:
    - Mean arterial pressure
    - Arterial PO_2
    - Arterial PCO_2
    - Cerebral metabolic rate
    - Body temperature
    - Anesthetic agents – volatiles, ketamine, propofol

7. There is approximately 150 mL of CSF, which is in constant circulation from brain to spinal cord. It is produced in the choroid plexuses of the lateral, third and fourth ventricles at a rate of around 500 mL/24 hr. It passes from the lateral ventricle to the third ventricle via the foramina of Munro, from the third to fourth ventricle via the Sylvian aqueduct and leaves the fourth ventricle through the foramina of Luschka laterally and foramen of Magendie medially. It is absorbed by the arachnoid villi, mainly in the brain, but it is also absorbed via the spinal arachnoid villi.

7 Coronary Circulation

Candidate's Instructions

Look at the following two diagrams. Label them appropriately and answer the questions.

(a)

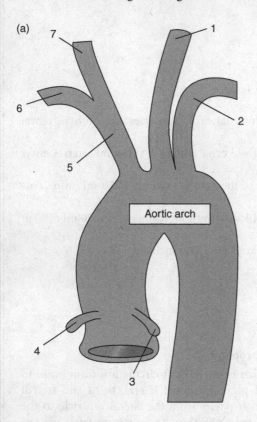

Aortic arch

Adapted from Gray H. *Gray's Anatomy*. 1918. Image in the public domain.

Questions

1. Label the branches of the aorta (1–7).

(b)

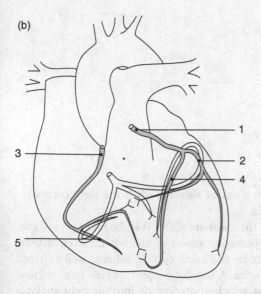

Erdmann A. *Concise Anatomy for Anaesthesia*. Cambridge. 2007. Reproduced with permission.

2. Name the vessels 1–5.
3. Where do the left and right coronary arteries arise from?
4. Describe the venous drainage of the heart?
5. What is the innervation of the heart?
6. What signs and symptoms might arise from reduced blood flow to the right coronary artery?

Answers

1. 1. Left common carotid artery
   2. Left subclavian artery
   3. Left coronary artery
   4. Right coronary artery
   5. Brachiocephalic trunk
   6. Right subclavian artery
   7. Right common carotid artery
2. 1. Left main coronary artery
   2. Circumflex artery
   3. Right coronary artery
   4. Left anterior descending artery
   5. Right marginal branch
3. The left coronary artery arises from the left sinus of Valsalva while the right coronary artery arises from the right sinus of Valsalva.
4. The majority of venous drainage occurs via the coronary sinus. It is the main vein of the myocardium running left to right in the posterior aspect of the left atrioventricular groove. It receives blood from the great, middle and small cardiac veins as well as from the left marginal and posterior ventricular veins. A smaller percentage (20–30%) occurs via the anterior cardiac and Thebesian veins, which drain directly into the right atrium.
5. The innervation of the heart is via the autonomic nervous system from superficial and deep cardiac plexuses. The sympathetic supply is from presynaptic fibers of T1–T5 and postsynaptic fibers from the cervical sympathetic chain ganglia. The parasympathetic supply is derived from the vagus nerve.
6. The right coronary artery supplies the right atrium and ventricle (in the majority of people) as well as some of the posterior wall of the left ventricle and the anterior two-thirds of the interventricular septum. The right coronary artery also supplies much of the conducting system of the heart. Reduced blood flow will result in ischemia to that area. The symptoms range from nothing to general malaise, sweating, fatigue and nausea and may progress to the classical symptoms of chest pain and shortness of breath. Signs would include anxiety, tachycardia, arrhythmias, hypotension, pulmonary edema and tachypnea. Bradycardia and heart block can also be seen as the sinus node and the atrioventricular bundle are usually vascularized by branches of the right coronary artery.

The vasculature of the aorta and coronary vessels is bread-and-butter cardiac anatomy and has major clinical relevance to anesthesia. You may get angiograms to look at in this station as well as diagrams and models of the heart.

8 Base of Skull

Candidate's Instructions

This station will test your knowledge of cranial anatomy.

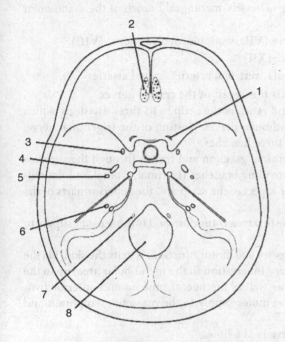

Erdmann A. *Concise Anatomy for Anaesthesia*. Cambridge. 2007. Reproduced with permission.

Questions

1. Label the canals/foramina 1–8 and state which nerves pass through them.
2. How would you test trigeminal nerve function?
3. What are the functions of cranial nerve VII?

Answers

1. 1. Optic canal: optic nerve (II), ophthalmic artery, sympathetic nerves
   2. Cribriform plate: olfactory nerve (I)
   3. Foramen rotundum: maxillary division of the trigeminal nerve (V)
   4. Foramen ovale: mandibular branch of the trigeminal nerve (V), accessory meningeal artery
   5. Foramen spinosum: middle meningeal vessels, meningeal branch of the mandibular nerve
   6. Internal auditory meatus: facial nerve (VII), vestibulocochlear nerve (VIII)
   7. Hypoglossal canal: hypoglossal nerve (XII)
   8. Foramen magnum: medulla oblongata, vertebral arteries, spinal arteries

2. The trigeminal nerve (cranial nerve V) is the largest of the cranial nerves.

   It provides sensory supply to the face and much of the scalp in its three divisions, which are the ophthalmic, maxillary and mandibular nerves. Testing of the trigeminal nerve, therefore, requires assessment of these three branches.

   The ophthalmic branch leaves the trigeminal ganglion and travels through the superior orbital fissure. It is a sensory nerve, providing branches (lacrimal, frontal and nasociliary) to supply sensation to the anterior aspect of the scalp and the superior parts of the face, including the cornea.

   The maxillary branch passes through the foramen rotundum and is the sensory supply to the mid-face.

   The mandibular branch has a mixed sensory and motor function. It exits the skull via the foramen ovale. It has an extensive sensory innervation to the mandibular area, up to the temporomandibular joint and temple as well as the buccal mucosa and anterior two-thirds of the tongue. It also provides the motor supply to the masseter, temporalis and pterygoid muscles.

   Therefore, testing of the trigeminal nerve is as follows:

   - Test for light touch, pin-prick and temperature in the three separate nerve distributions
   - Test the corneal reflex (motor response via the facial nerve)
   - Ask the patient to clench his/her jaw and palpate the masseter and temporalis muscles for volume and tone
   - Open the mouth and observe for mandibular deviation
   - Test lateral jaw movement against resistance

3. The facial nerve has motor and sensory functions. It exits the skull via the internal auditory meatus along with the vestibulocochlear nerve (VIII).

   It is the motor to most of the facial muscles, notably the frontalis, orbicularis oculi, orbicularis oris, platysma and stapedius. Therefore, it is involved in providing innervation for blinking, frowning and smiling.

   Its sensory component is responsible for taste to the anterior two-thirds of the tongue; it also has a secretory function to the lacrimal gland, nose and mouth, and submandibular and sublingual salivary glands.

   As well as being able to identify the different foramina, you need to know the structures they transmit. This knowledge may be tested in asking about specific signs and symptoms relating to intracranial pathologies.

9 Diaphragm

Candidate's Instructions

Look at the given diagram and answer the following questions.

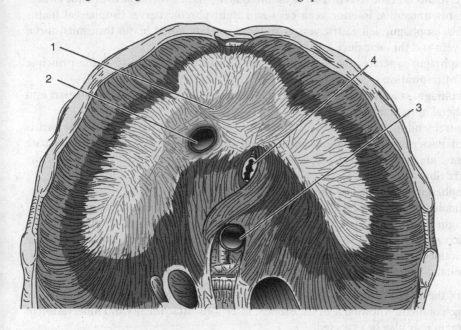

Adapted from Gray H. *Gray's Anatomy*. 1918. Image in the public domain.

Questions

1. Label structures 1–4.
2. At what levels are the three diaphragmatic foramina?
3. What does each of them transmit?
4. What is the function of the diaphragm?
5. What is it composed of?
6. What are its attachments?
7. What is its nerve supply?
8. What is a Bochdalek hernia?

Answers

1. 1. Central tendon of the diaphragm
   2. Inferior vena cava (IVC) hiatus
   3. Aorta/aortic hiatus
   4. Esophagus/esophageal hiatus
2. The IVC hiatus is at the level of T8; the esophageal hiatus at T10; the aortic hiatus at T12.
3. IVC hiatus transmits: inferior vena cava and right phrenic nerve. Esophageal hiatus transmits: esophagus, left gastric vessels and vagus nerve. Aortic hiatus transmits: aorta, azygos vein and thoracic duct.
4. The diaphragm separates the abdominal cavity from the thorax and is the principle muscle of respiration.
5. The diaphragm is a sheet of skeletal muscle composed of a central tendinous part and a peripheral muscular part.
6. The central tendon is in contact with the pericardium superiorly. The muscular part is attached posteriorly to the psoas muscle and quadratus lumborum via the arcuate ligaments, medially to the xiphisternum and anteriorly to the costal cartilages of the lower six ribs.
7. The diaphragm is supplied by the phrenic nerve (C3, C4 and C5).
8. A Bochdalek hernia is a type of congenital diaphragmatic hernia. Disruption of the diaphragm during fetal development allows the abdominal viscera to push into the thoracic cavity. It can cause pulmonary hypertension and hypoplastic lungs, resulting in respiratory distress of the newborn.
   Congenital diaphragmatic hernia carries a mortality rate of 35–60 percent.

The crux of the station is in knowing the different foramina, their levels and what passes through each of them. Knowledge of the origins, insertions, attachments and innervation of the diaphragm may also be expected.

10 Spinal Cord

Candidate's Instructions

A cross-section of the spinal cord is shown here. Please answer the following questions.

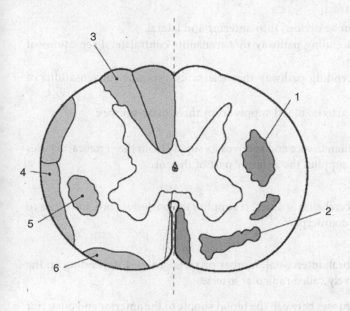

Erdmann A. *Concise Anatomy for Anaesthesia*. Cambridge. 2007. Reproduced with permission.

Questions

1. Label structures 1–6.
2. What are the functions of the spinothalamic tracts?
3. What is the blood supply to the spinal cord?
4. What is the artery of Adamkiewicz?
5. What is its venous drainage?
6. What is anterior spinal artery syndrome?
7. How many pairs of spinal nerves are there?
8. What are the anterior primary rami?
9. What are the features of spinal shock?

Answers

1. 1. Lateral corticospinal tract
    2. Vestibulospinal tract
    3. Fasciculus cuneatus
    4. Posterior spinocerebellar tract
    5. Lateral spinothalamic tract
    6. Anterior spinothalamic tract

2. The spinothalamic tracts can be divided into anterior and lateral.
   Anterior spinothalamic – ascending pathway that transmits contralateral sensations of touch and pressure.
   Lateral spinothalamic – ascending pathway that transmits contralateral sensations of pain and temperature.

3. The spinal cord receives its arterial blood supply from three main sources:
   - *Anterior spinal artery*
   This lies on the anterior median fissure and receives its supply from the vertebral arteries at the foramen magnum. It supplies the anterior part of the cord

   - *Posterior spinal artery*
   Formed from the posterior cerebellar arteries. It supplies the posterior cord and tends to be smaller than its anterior counterpart

   - *Other spinal arteries*
   These are branches of vertebral, intercostal, lumbar or sacral arteries, depending on the cord level. They are collectively called radicular arteries

   - There are few/no anastomoses between the blood supply to the anterior and posterior cord. This leaves those areas vulnerable to ischemia from disruption to the anterior or posterior spinal arteries (e.g. thrombosis, spasm and hypotension).

4. The artery of Adamkiewicz (named after a Polish pathologist), also known as the arteria radicularis magna, is one of the radicular arteries arising from the lower thoracic region. It is of importance because it has a major role in the blood supply to the lower half of the spinal cord.

5. Venous drainage of the spinal cord is via lateral, anterior and posterior venous plexuses. They unite to drain into larger regional vessels such as the azygos, vertebral, lumbar and sacral veins.

6. Anterior spinal artery syndrome results from infarction or ischemia of the anterior spinal artery. It presents with paralysis and loss of pain and temperature sensation below the level of the insult. Proprioception is usually preserved.

7. There are 31 pairs of spinal nerves – 8 cervical, 12 thoracic, 5 lumbar, 5 sacral and 1 coccygeal.

8. The anterior primary rami give cutaneous and motor supply to the limbs and the anterior and lateral parts of the neck, thorax and abdomen.
   The posterior primary rami give sensory and motor supply to the muscles and skin of the back.

9. Spinal shock occurs following injury to the spinal cord. It initially presents with loss of sensory and motor function below the level of the lesion; it may be accompanied by

hypotension and bradycardia, depending on the level of the injury, due to disruption of sympathetic tone. Following the initial period of hyporeflexia, some reflexes will return over the next week or so with a period of hyperreflexia appearing within the following four to six weeks. Roughly six weeks following injury, there may be evidence of hyper-reflexia and spasticity as well as autonomic dysfunction.

Autonomic dysreflexia is a condition associated with spinal cord injury that usually results from cord injury above the level of T6. It can result in extreme hypertension, compensatory bradycardia, flushing, sweating and headaches. It is often triggered by painful stimuli below the level of the cord lesion.

There is a wealth of relevant information the examiner can quiz you on. It may involve labelling a cross-section of the spinal cord and a more in-depth discussion surrounding the functions of various tracts. You may also be asked about the effects of cord transsection or signs and symptoms of various spinal cord lesions.

11 Wrist

Candidate's Instructions

This station is based around the anatomy and regional anesthesia of the wrist.

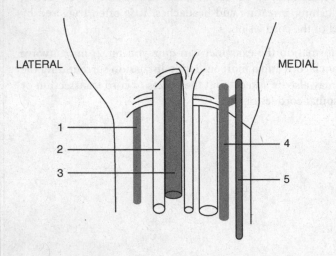

Questions

1. Label structures 1–5.
2. What is the motor and sensory distribution of the ulnar nerve?
3. Describe the origin of the radial nerve and its course in the forearm.
4. What is the sensory distribution of the radial nerve in the hand?
5. What is Allen's test?
6. What are the indications for a wrist block?
7. Describe the landmark technique for blocking the median and ulnar nerves?
8. What are the complications of wrist blocks?

Answers

1. 1. Radial artery
   2. Flexor carpi radialis
   3. Median nerve
   4. Ulnar artery
   5. Ulnar nerve

2. The ulnar nerve gives its motor supply to the majority of the intrinsic muscles of the hand, which includes all the interossei, adductor pollicis, the three hypothenar muscles and the medial two lumbricals. The rest (LOAF) are supplied by the median nerve.
   (LOAF – lateral two lumbricals, opponens pollicis, abductor pollicis brevis and flexor pollicis brevis.
   The sensory distribution of the ulnar nerve is over the medial one and a half digits.)

3. The radial nerve is the largest branch of the brachial plexus; it is derived from the spinal nerves of C5 to T1.
   The radial nerve enters the forearm and divides into deep and superficial branches. The superficial branch passes under the cover of the brachioradialis muscle to emerge in the distal part of the forearm where it passes over the top of the anatomical snuff box.
   The deep branch, a direct continuation of the radial nerve, pierces the supinator muscle to enter the posterior compartment of the forearm, travelling laterally down towards the wrist.

4. The radial nerve supplies no muscles in the hand. It is purely sensory and supplies the skin over the lateral two-thirds of the dorsum of the hand, thumb and the proximal parts of the lateral one and a half digits.

5. Allen's test is used to check for collateral arterial blood supply to the hand. It may be used when taking arterial blood gases or inserting an arterial line. It involves holding the forearm upright, occluding both the radial and ulnar arteries at the wrist and then releasing the ulnar artery while continuing to compress the radial artery. If collateral blood supply exists, the hand should go pink as the ulnar artery perfuses the radial aspect of the hand.

6. A wrist block may be used for surgery of the hand and fingers.

7. *Median nerve* – insert a needle between the tendons of flexor carpi radialis and palmaris longus (there may be a "pop" as you pass through fascia) and then inject 4–6 mL of local anesthetic.
   Ulnar nerve – insert a needle just above the styloid process and under the tendon of the flexor carpi ulnaris. Pass 0.5 cm under the tendon and inject 4–6 mL of local anesthetic.

8. Complications of wrist blocks include:
   - Patient discomfort on injection
   - Failure
   - Infection
   - Nerve damage
   - Hematoma
   - Intravascular injection
   - Damage to insensate digits following surgery

12 Larynx

Candidate's Instructions

Please look at this model/diagram of the larynx and answer the following questions.

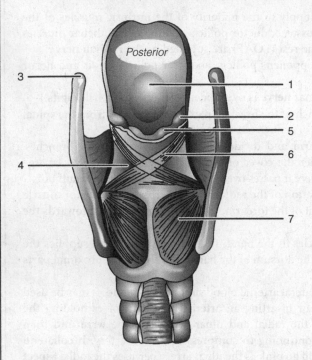

Posterior

3
1
2
5
6
4
7

Adapted from Gray H. *Gray's Anatomy*. 1918. Image in the public domain.

Questions

1. Label structures 1–7.
2. Name the main intrinsic muscles of the larynx and describe their functions.
3. What is the blood supply to the larynx?
4. What is the nerve supply to the larynx?
5. At what vertebral level is the thyroid notch?
6. When can the recurrent laryngeal nerve be damaged?
7. What is the clinical difference between unilateral and bilateral recurrent laryngeal nerve damage?

Answers

1. 1. Epiglottis
    2. Cuneiform cartilage
    3. Superior horn (cornu) of the thyroid cartilage
    4. Oblique arytenoid muscle (part of the interarytenoid muscles)
    5. Corniculate cartilage
    6. Transverse arytenoid muscle (other part of the interarytenoid muscles)
    7. Posterior cricoarytenoid muscle
2. The intrinsic muscles of the larynx are responsible for:
    *   Altering the tension of the vocal cords to allow speech
    *   Opening the vocal cords during inspiration
    *   Closing the vocal cords during swallowing

    The intrinsic muscles of the larynx are:
    *   Posterior cricoarytenoid: abducts the cords, opens the glottis
    *   Lateral cricoarytenoid: adducts the cords, closes the glottis
    *   Interarytenoid muscles: close the glottis
    *   Thyroarytenoid: relaxes cord tension
    *   Vocalis: acts to adjust the tension in the vocal cords
    *   Cricothyroid: regulates cord tension
3. The larynx receives its blood supply from the superior and inferior laryngeal arteries. The *superior laryngeal artery* is a branch of the superior thyroid artery, from the external carotid. It pierces the thyrohyoid membrane to supply the interior of the larynx. The *inferior laryngeal artery* is a branch of the inferior thyroid artery, from the subclavian artery. It lies close to the recurrent laryngeal nerve in its passage to the larynx.
4. The nerve supply to the larynx is from branches of the vagus nerve.

    The *superior laryngeal nerve* divides into a small external branch and a larger internal branch. The external branch is the motor supply to the cricothyroid muscle. The internal branch pierces the thyrohyoid membrane with the superior laryngeal artery. It provides sensory innervation of the larynx down to the vocal cords, as well as of the inferior surface of the epiglottis.

    The *recurrent laryngeal nerve* has a slightly different course on each side. On the right, it leaves the vagus and loops under the subclavian artery and then ascends in the tracheo-esophageal groove. The left recurrent laryngeal nerve loops under the aortic arch and then also ascends in the (left) tracheoesophageal groove. It supplies the motor component for all the intrinsic muscles of the larynx except for cricothyroid. It also provides the sensory supply to the larynx below the vocal cords.
5. The thyroid notch lies at the level of C4.

    The hyoid bone lies around C3 while the cricoid cartilage lies at the level of C5.
6. The recurrent laryngeal nerve is classically at risk of damage during thyroid surgery as it lies directly posterior to the gland. It may also be damaged by a goiter, enlarged lymph nodes or cervical trauma. The left recurrent laryngeal nerve is also at risk from malignant mediastinal tumors or even aortic aneurysms (or ascending aortic or arch surgery) because of its course.

7. Unilateral damage commonly results in hoarseness due to impaired movement of the affected cord and a midline position.

Bilateral damage can lead to aphonia and stridor with airway obstruction because of a total loss of vocal cord function.

Further Reading List

Abrahams PH, Hutchings RT, Marks SC. *McMinn's Colour Atlas of Human Anatomy.* Mosby, 1998.

Erdmann A. *Concise Anatomy for Anaesthesia.* Cambridge University Press, 2007.

Gray H. *Gray's Anatomy.* Running Press, 1974.

Moore KL, Dalley AF. *Clinically Oriented Anatomy.* Lippincott Williams and Wilkins, 1992.

Open Anesthesia Anatomy (ABA). See www.openanesthesia.org /laryngeal_innervation/

Introduction

History taking is a core skill for every medical professional and is something that has been drilled into all of us since our first day at medical school. It is of vital importance to take an accurate, detailed and clear history when seeing any patient prior to anesthesia. In clinical practice, this can sometimes be difficult due to time constraints, finding appropriate notes, waiting for patients to arrive, etc. In the examination, some of these issues will not be a problem; however, time really is against you.

A common misconception is to think "I take anesthetic histories every day; I do not need to practice this." Wrong. Without practice you may fail this station.

In the history-taking station you will be presented with a patient who is likely to be undergoing surgery and you are there to take an appropriate history. It can be quite a challenge to get all the points necessary in such a short period of time, so before entering the station you must have a systematic, stepwise approach to your history taking. It is hard to know if points are going to be awarded for finding out the intricacies of why they are presenting for surgery or for knowledge about an unrelated medical problem. You will almost certainly gain points for introducing yourself, checking the patient's identity and communicating clearly. It may sound simple but forget to do these things and you have lost three points before you have even started.

If the patient is having surgery, you will need to focus some of your time on the relevant body system; for example, for thyroid surgery you will be expected to ask about the signs and symptoms of thyroid disease as well as effects on the airway and any anesthetic problems it may cause.

There are also some questions specific to an anesthetic history that every anesthesiologist should ask during the preoperative visit. Again, these points are extremely important and, if you miss them out, you will throw away easy points; you do it every day so do it in the examination!

In this chapter, we will go through a widely practiced approach to history taking, then focus on some of the more pertinent points you should ask regarding the different body systems and, finally, finish with a few scenarios. Admittedly, the scenarios are by no means a comprehensive guide to all the possible cases you may face in the examination but they cover some of the more common topics and contain potential patient questions and candidate responses. The scenarios are to be used as a framework that you may wish to expand on or go through with a colleague. Rehearse your history-taking system, communicate effectively, ask the questions specific to an anesthetic history and you will nail it. An appropriate order for history taking is:

- Introduction
- History of presenting complaint
- Past medical history
- Past surgical history
- Systems review
- Drug history and allergies
- Social history

- Family history
- Anesthesia specific questions

Introduction

It is always important to make a good first impression on examiners, so politely introduce yourself to the patient and start with a few housekeeping questions:

- Confirm the patient's identity
- If they are having surgery, confirm what it is and which side (if applicable)
- Then start with an opening comment such as "I need to ask you a few questions regarding . . .," or along similar lines
- Do this **quickly** and **confidently** and you will put the patient and yourself at ease

History of Presenting Complaint

It is important to ask why the patient is having the procedure done as this may give clues as to further questions you may need to ask; for instance, a cystoscopy may be for suspected malignancy or before urethrotomy; in each case, further lines of questioning will be different.

Start with an open question – "Can you tell me about the problems you've been having that have resulted in you needing this surgery?" Then fill in any blanks with some closed questions to save time.

Past Medical History

This can be ascertained by asking a simple open question such as "Do you have any medical complaints or problems?" or "Do you see a doctor for any medical issues?" In real life, some patients are not overly forthcoming with information but, in the OSCE, if you ask this they are obliged to tell you. Any illnesses missed out can be covered in the systems review, which you **must** do. In addition, remember to ask if they have had any medical problems or serious illnesses in the past that are not being treated currently. Take note of any problems they tell you about and be sure to explore each medical problem fully.

Past Surgical History

In a similar fashion, you should ask about any previous surgery. You need to know the type of surgery and when it was. A simple question like "Have you had any operations in the past?" will suffice.

This may give you a clue as to how well they have tolerated anesthesia in the past and also provide important information about the body system involved. If they have had spinal surgery, it may make spinal anesthesia difficult; previous surgery to the airway may increase the likelihood of a difficult intubation; nephrectomy will have a bearing on drugs used, and drug doses, and so on.

Systems Review

This is usually done alongside the past medical history. By asking questions on each of the major different body systems, you ensure that you are not missing any important medical information.

If the patient gives a positive response to any of these questions then carefully explore the problem again.

A few quick questions from each category will usually suffice and can be modified into a list style of questioning to save time. You must be able to rattle these off without having to think too hard about them.

Cardiovascular

- Have you ever had a heart attack/palpitations/ankle swelling/chest pains/shortness of breath (at rest or on exertion)?
- Exercise tolerance and activities of daily living

Respiratory

- Have you ever suffered with any chest problems such as asthma or chronic obstructive pulmonary disease (COPD)?
- Do you have a long-standing cough/wheeze/sputum-production problems?
- Have you ever used or do you use any inhalers?

Musculoskeletal and Central Nervous System (CNS)

- Do you suffer with joint pain? Arthritis?
- Do you have epilepsy? Have you ever had a stroke?
- Do you suffer with headaches or migraines?
- Have you ever had a blackout? Seizures?

Genitourinary and Gastrointestinal

- Any constipation/loose stool, swallowing problems, reflux or weight loss?
- Any frequency, dysuria, nocturia or hesitancy?
- Dysmenorrhea, intermenstrual bleeding, last menstrual period (LMP)?

Drug History and Allergies

Always ask **first** about any **allergies** and that way you will not forget. If the patient does have an allergy, ask how it presents itself – is it a rash, full-blown anaphylaxis, or something else?

Take as detailed a drug history as time will allow and try to remember to ask about the contraceptive pill (commonly forgotten). This may be particularly relevant if there are coexisting risk factors for deep vein thrombosis (DVT) and pulmonary embolism (PE) or if you will administer aprepitant (Emend), which lowers the efficacy of hormonally based contraception (pills, patches, and some implants and intrauterine devices (IUDs).

Social History

Ask the patient if he/she smokes and, if so, how many per day and for how long. If he/she has stopped, ask when. Ask if the patient drinks alcohol and how much per week.

A couple of points that people often forget is to ask about recreational drug use and, if the patient is female of childbearing age, you should ask if there is a chance she may be pregnant.

Family History

Be sure to ask about any medical problems that run in the family and if there are any problems with general anesthesia. Explore the patient's answer fully as it poses the possibility of pseudocholinesterase deficiency or malignant hyperthermia, which could be a whole station in itself. Ask if the person has had the appropriate tests if you think it is a possibility.

Anesthetic Specific Questions

A useful tip is to try and cover these questions at the start of the session as you may either forget at the end or run out of time and you will lose points for not asking them as they are very important.

You must ask about:

- Previous anesthetics and any problems – postoperative nausea and vomiting (PONV), wake-up (emergence), difficult airway, etc.
- Family history (see earlier)
- Dentition – caps, crowns, loose teeth, dentures
- Symptoms of reflux and heartburn
- Neck problems or stiffness
- Ability to take nonsteroidal anti-inflammatory drugs, acetaminophen and gabapentin
- Have they met NPO preoperative fasting guidelines if the procedure is that day

Be **confident** and **attentive** when taking the history and you will do well.

We will now look at some body systems and pathologies that patients may present with. Along with each problem are some suggested questions to ask in order to ascertain how serious or significant the disease is.

Cardiovascular

Hypertension

- How long has the patient had hypertension?
- How well controlled is the blood pressure (BP)? Does the patient know his/her normal BP or even check it at home?
- What medications does the patient take for it? How compliant is he/she with treatment? Has he/she experienced any side effects from the medication; for example, dry cough with an angiotensin converting enzyme (ACE) inhibitor?
- Does the patient see his/her physician regularly about it?
- Are there any long-standing effects? Is there evidence of end organ damage such as renal impairment, visual impairment, coronary artery disease?

Ischemic Heart Disease

- How long for? What medications? How compliant is the patient with treatment?
- Does the patient get chest pain? If so when, at rest or on exertion? Does he/she use nitroglycerin and how often does he/she need to use it?
- How far can the patient walk? Does he/she get short of breath? If so when?
- Can the patient lie flat at night? Is there ankle swelling or other signs of heart failure?

- Has the patient ever had a myocardial infarct (MI)? Any history of cardiac surgery? Is he/she under the care of a cardiologist?

Valvular Heart Disease

- Which valve(s) is/are affected? How long? What treatment? Is the patient on any anticoagulant therapy?
- Any investigations? Valve replacement surgery? Cardiology opinion? Recent echocardiogram? Any previous anesthetic issues?
- Is the patient symptomatic; that is, blackouts, shortness of breath, arrhythmias or chest pain? Presence of symptomatic valvular heart disease places a patient in a high-risk group for perioperative complications

Pacemakers

- What type of pacemaker is it? When and why was it inserted?
- Is the patient followed? Has the pacemaker been checked recently? What mode and rate?
- Is there a recent ECG available? Has the patient ever had any problems with the pacemaker?

Respiratory

COPD or Asthma

- How long has the patient suffered with it? What treatments are taken and how often? How compliant is the patient? Does he/she take steroids?
- What is the patient's exercise tolerance? What are his/her peak flow readings? Does he/she get breathless or have dyspnea? If so, when (activity level)?
- How severe is the disease? How often does the patient have attacks? Does he/she see a physician regularly for it? Has the patient ever had any hospital admissions with it? If so, has he/she been admitted to the intensive care unit as a result?
- Does the patient need home oxygen? Is he/she under the care of a respiratory physician?
- Has the patient had any investigations such as pulmonary function tests, CT scans, etc.?
- Can the patient lie flat? How many pillows does he/she sleep with (orthopnea)?
- Enquire about smoking status and document specific allergies and any intolerance to nonsteroidal anti-inflammatory drugs (NSAIDs)

Note: for COPD, try and include some cardiac questions as well because there may be coexisting disease.

Musculoskeletal

Arthritis

- How long has the patient suffered with arthritis? How severe is it? Which joints are most affected?
- What treatments does the patient take? Is he/she compliant with medication? Take a detailed drug history

- Is it osteoarthritis (OA) or rheumatoid arthritis (RA)? There may be more complications associated with RA such as anemia, pulmonary nodules, atlantoaxial subluxation and the use of steroids and associated side effects
- What is the patient's neck range of motion? Does it affect jaw opening? Does he/she have any spinal or big joint deformities?
- How much does it affect the patient's daily activities? How far can he/she walk? If the patient cannot walk far, is it a result of the arthritis or some other pathology such as heart failure or COPD?

CNS disorders

Epilepsy

- When was the patient diagnosed? What type of epilepsy is it? How frequent is it? What medications does he/she take? When was his/her last seizure?
- Does the patient hold a driver's license? To what extent does epilepsy affect his/her lifestyle?

Parkinson's Disease

- How long has the patient had Parkinson's disease? What medications does he/she take? Any brain implant? Is he/she under the care of a neurologist? How severe is it? You will need a detailed drug history
- How regular is the patient's medication? He/she may need replacement via a nasogastric tube intraoperatively if it is to be a long procedure
- Is there a history of dysphagia or reflux (significant aspiration risk)?
- Are there any concerns over respiratory function? To what extent is the patient's activity restricted?

Endocrine

Thyroid Disease

- Ascertain if this is hypo- or hyperthyroidism as you will need to ask about signs and symptoms accordingly
- How long has the patient had the problem? What treatment is he/she on? What medications have been tried in the past? What symptoms does he/she complain of?
- Has the patient had any adverse effects of therapy so far? Is he/she looked after by an endocrinologist?
- If hypothyroid, ask about weight gain, cold intolerance, bradycardia and any neck swelling
- If hyperthyroid, ask about palpitations, tremor, restlessness, arrhythmias, weight loss, diarrhea, exophthalmos and neck swelling
- If the patient is having surgery on the neck, ask why. Have other treatments failed? Has he/she previously had surgery on the neck? Is there a mass or swelling? If so, you **must** ask about stridor, change in voice, any difficulty or alterations in breathing. Are there any symptoms of airway obstruction? Can the patient lie flat without a problem? Are there any swallowing difficulties?
- Does the patient have any other autoimmune conditions?

Diabetes Mellitus

- How long has he/she had it? What medications does he/she take? When was the last dose of metformin? Is the patient insulin dependent? What is the patient's compliance? Does he/she monitor his/her blood sugars regularly?
- Does the patient know his/her HbA1c?
- Does the patient often have hypoglycemic episodes? Has he/she ever been admitted to hospital? Does he/she have any current infections?
- Has the patient developed any small vessel disease such as neuropathy, nephropathy and retinopathy?
- Does the patient have coexisting vascular disease such as ischemic heart disease, hypertension or intermittent claudication?
- Has the patient ever had a stroke or an MI? Does he/she have hyperlipidemia? Does the patient have any other autoimmune conditions?
- Does he/she have any gastrointestinal symptoms? They can have delayed gastric emptying as part of an autonomic dysfunction and may need longer NPO times before surgery. Many diabetics are prone to reflux as a result of gastroparesis

1 TURP Surgery

Candidate's Instructions and Questions

You are instructed to take a history from an 82-year-old gentleman who has been scheduled for a palliative (non-curative) transurethral resection of the prostate (TURP).

1. How will you start the history?

   He tells you that it is for recurring prostate cancer and that he has osteoarthritis (OA) and chronic obstructive pulmonary disease (COPD).

2. What questions will you ask him now and what is of importance to the history?

   On a systems review, he discloses that he has an irregular heartbeat that is looked after by his cardiologist.

3. What else will you need to know and look at?

   You get a good drug history but he is allergic to the antibiotic that was used last time.

4. What is important to ask and how will you find out what antibiotic it is?
5. What anesthetic specific questions do you need to ask?

   He tells you he had an injection in his back for the same procedure two years ago but there was some difficulty.

6. How would you approach this?

Answers

This type of patient is not uncommon on urology schedules and getting a full history can be difficult but is of great importance.

1. Start as always by:
   - Introducing yourself
   - Confirming the patient's identity and the proposed procedure
   - Ask why he is having the procedure done
   - Obtain a history of the presenting problem
   - Then move onto his past medical and surgical history
2. You have managed to ascertain why he is having the procedure and that he has the described comorbidities. It may be pertinent to ask about urinary symptoms as well as stigmata of metastatic prostate cancer, but do not focus too much on these unless they are offered up. Ask about his OA: how long has he had it, the joints affected, how it limits his lifestyle, any joint replacements, range of movements (particularly neck and back). Regarding his COPD, ask what medication he takes, how long has he had it, what treatments he takes, how often he uses his inhalers, if he takes steroids, how severe it is, if he has any investigations, any hospital admissions and what his exercise tolerance is like. Does he smoke or has he ever smoked? Again try and include a few cardiovascular screening questions at this stage as well.
3. Having done the systems review, you realize he is likely to have atrial fibrillation (A Fib).
   - Get a more detailed history
   - When and how was this discovered? What exactly is he taking for it? Is he taking anticoagulants? Is he aware of palpitations? How does it affect him?
   - You will certainly need to look at an ECG and recent blood test results, including an international normalized ratio (INR) if he's taking warfarin (Coumadin). Most patients having this procedure will have a complete blood count (CBC), basic electrolyte analysis, blood urea nitrogen and creatinine
4. You need to find out what type of reaction he had to the antibiotic.
   - He tells you it caused a rash that disappeared the next day
   - You will find the information on the previous anesthetic chart or in his preoperative notes
5. Every history should include these anesthetic specific questions:
   - Any previous anesthetics, including family, and any problems that occurred?
   - Any dentition issues – dentures, caps, crowns, bridges?
   - Any symptoms of acid reflux or indigestion?
   - Any neck problems (already established, hopefully, in asking about his arthritis). When was his last food and drink?
   - Is he able to take nonsteroidal anti-inflammatory drugs (NSAIDs) (although sometimes not asked in the elderly as age and compounding renal impairment would prevent its administration)?
   - Do not forget to ask about smoking, alcohol and drug use
6. The patient is, of course, referring to a spinal anesthetic and, with increasing age and OA, it may be difficult to insert a spinal needle. Again, look at the previous anesthetic record to identify what problems were encountered. You could try the lateral position if sitting is difficult for him and see at which space the subarachnoid space was found previously. If the previous attempt used the midline approach, you could try a paramedian approach.

Reassure the patient and suggest that general anesthesia may have to be the alternative, if spinal anesthesia is difficult.

Remember this is a history-taking station, so don't waste time obtaining consent for a spinal or general anesthesia.

2 Laparoscopic Cholecystectomy

Candidate's Instructions and Questions

"This is Mr. Oswald and he is due to have a laparoscopic cholecystectomy this week. He has attended a preoperative clinic. Can you take a relevant history?"

1. How do you proceed?

He says he has had problems with his gallbladder for years but surgeons have been reluctant to do anything because of his weight. His past medical history includes diabetes mellitus and hypertension.

2. What line of questioning will you follow now?

He tells you he is about 336 pounds, and his blood pressure is well controlled. His blood sugars are usually of no concern and he has never been admitted to hospital. Further questioning reveals that he is tired during the day and his partner sleeps in a separate room.

3. Are there any other symptoms you need to ask about?

Having taken a drug history, you learn from him that his medications are atorvastatin, amlodipine and his internist has just started him on insulin.

4. What do you need to know now?
5. What anesthetic-specific questions do you need to ask?

He states he has had previous general anesthesia without any problems but suffers from reflux.

6. Is there anything else you would ask, knowing this?

Answers

Individuals in the general population are getting bigger and this can mean more challenging surgery and anesthesia. Be sure to explore every avenue when taking a history from someone with a high body mass index (BMI).

1. Again, start introducing yourself, checking patient identity and asking relevant questions around the proposed procedure. Follow this up with a detailed past medical and surgical history.

2. Obviously, if the male patient has a high BMI, this will be clear when you meet him; it is important to ask if he knows his height and weight. Sensitively ask about problems regarding the patient's weight such as how it affects his mobility, is he active, does it affect any joints? In this particular case, explore why surgeons have decided to operate now: has he lost weight, is it affecting his daily living to a greater extent? Regarding his hypertension, what medications does he take, how well controlled is it, how long has he been on treatment and is he compliant? Regarding his diabetes; is he type 1 or type 2, how long has he been diabetic, what medications is he on, is he compliant with treatment and what his blood sugars are like, are there any issues of small vessel disease and is his renal function normal?

3. You will need to explore this in a bit more detail. In this case, the history is suggestive of obstructive sleep apnea. You should ask about:
   STOP BANG Questionnaire
   - Snoring at night
   - Tired during the day
   - Observed to stop breathing at night
   - Blood Pressure
   - BMI greater than 35 kg/m^2
   - Age over 50 years old
   - Neck circumference greater than 40 cm
   - Gender male
   - If he has ever been investigated for sleep apnea
   - Postsurgery, this may have an impact on oxygen requirements and the need for continuous positive airway pressure (CPAP) overnight

4. You may well have asked about medications when you asked about his past medical history. However, it is useful for examination purposes to recap exactly what he is taking. He states he has just started on insulin – this is very important as it takes time for patients to get used to administering their own insulin and getting the dosage correct.
   You should ask why he was started on insulin, when it was started, whether he is established on a regimen currently, if he has had any hypoglycemic events and whether he is compliant with therapy. What is his HbA1c?

5. Do not forget to ask the anesthetic specific questions detailed previously.

6. Reassuringly, he has had a previous general anesthetic, but ask how big he was then. Clarify how bad his reflux is as this will affect your management. You should ask whether he takes antacids, H2 blockers or proton pump inhibitors, gets reflux all the time, and if he has actual acid regurgitation or "heartburn"-like symptoms.

3 Thyroid Surgery

Candidate's Instructions and Questions

You are instructed to take a preoperative history from a 53-year-old lady who is having thyroid surgery.

1. How would you begin taking this history?
2. What important signs and symptoms would you ask about?

She tells you that the swelling has only appeared in the last 6–12 months; she has noticed a change in her voice and has become increasingly anxious. Otherwise, she says she is fit and well and had her wrist plated when she was 17 years old without any problems.

3. What would you be concerned about?
4. What other assessments are essential, given this history?

She has a limited past medical history but is a smoker of 30 pack-years and has been prescribed something for a fast heartbeat.

5. What medications are important to consider?
6. What anesthetic specific questions will you ask?

She states she has never had an anesthetic before but her brother had a really bad reaction to anesthetic when he had his shoulder surgery.

7. How would you approach this?

Answers

Thyroid surgery incorporates various procedures ranging from node biopsies to total thyroidectomy. Be sure to understand fully why the patient is having surgery.

1. Of course, introduce yourself, confirm patient identity and make sure the consent form has been signed. It is vital to ascertain the reason why the patient is having surgery. Is it for hyperthyroidism, removal of malignancy or further evaluation of a nodule? You will need to explore the history of the complaint. If there is a lump, how long has it been there, has it grown rapidly, is it painful, is it fixed, has she noticed any other symptoms, does it affect her airway? Has she had any previous therapy to the thyroid? Then continue with a full past medical and surgical history.

2. You will need to ask about stigmata of thyroid disease:
   - *Hyperthyroidism* – weight loss, tremor, heat intolerance, overexcitability and palpitations, anxiety, shortness of breath, chest pain, blurred vision, diarrhea, menstrual irregularity and skin thinning
   - *Hypothyroidism* – weight gain, lethargy, cool peripheries, depression, constipation, edema and dry skin

   You will need to ask about airway problems. Does the patient feel short of breath, is she able to lie flat comfortably, has she noticed a change in voice, is there any audible stridor, can she go about her daily activities, can she eat and drink normally? You may also wish to know if the patient has had any previous neck/thyroid surgery.

3. A change in the voice should start alarm bells ringing!
   - An alteration in the voice is an indication that the recurrent laryngeal nerve may be affected and can be associated with thyroid cancer. Infiltration of the airway is a possibility and needs serious consideration
   - Anxiety and palpitations are symptoms of hyperthyroidism and may suggest atrial fibrillation. You need to take a brief cardiac history: is she aware of palpitations, does she get chest pain, has she ever noticed irregular beats and is she on any medication?

4. As mentioned time and again, a detailed assessment of the airway is vital. You may, in real life, have access to CT or ultrasound scans, which can demonstrate airway compression or invasion, but be guided by clues in the history; stridor is a worrying sign. Key investigations include thyroid function tests, pulmonary function tests, chest X-rays (+/– lateral and thoracic inlet views), ECG, CT neck and thorax, and nasoendoscopy.

5. Important drugs used in treating hyperthyroidism are:
   - *Beta-blockers* – commonly propranolol; be aware of hypotension and bradycardia
   - *Methimazole* – can cause jaundice, rashes, nausea, itching and serious side effects such as bone-marrow suppression. This should not be prescribed in the first trimester of pregnancy due to the potential to cause fetal abnormalities
   - *Propylthiouracil* – common side effects include nausea and vomiting, hair loss, skin pigmentation and, rarely, agranulocytosis or liver failure. It is usually considered a second line drug to methimazole
   - *Corticosteroids* – used if there is an immune component of the hyperthyroidism, or in thyroid storm to decrease peripheral conversion of T4 to T3. (It will also treat any relative adrenal insufficiency caused by the hyperthyroidism)

6. Every history should include the previously mentioned anesthetic specific questions and, for women, you should ask about her last menstrual period or a pregnancy test.

7. This may come up as an entire communication scenario but, in the history, you will obviously need to ascertain what exactly is meant by this. This is of great importance if the patient has never had an anesthetic themselves. What was the reaction and what was the drug? Did the brother end up in intensive care? Most important of all is to know if you are dealing with a case of pseudocholisterase deficiency, leading to prolonged apnea, from succinylcholine or malignant hyperthermia and if the family members have had the appropriate investigations. Be sure to mention these specifically; sometimes the patient may say their relative was on a ventilator for a few hours. It may be a case of an allergic reaction to an antibiotic or muscle relaxant.

4 Shoulder Replacement

Candidate's Instructions and Questions

"This is Mrs. Wood – she is a 71-year-old lady who is scheduled for a shoulder replacement – please take an appropriate history."

1. How will you conduct your history taking?

   She tells you she has RA and her mobility is quite limited.

2. What should you pay particular interest to in the history?

   On systems review, she states she occasionally gets chest pain.

3. What further questions will you ask?
4. What medications would you be concerned about?

   She now remembers that she sees a cardiologist for her ischemic heart disease and, in the past, she has had renal problems with nonsteroidal anti-inflammatory drugs (NSAIDs).

5. What anesthetic specific questions will you ask?
6. What problems might you anticipate with such a patient?

   In a previous general anesthetic, they had difficulty intubating her and she says she has particular problems with her neck.

7. Is there anything else you would like to do?

Answers

1. Begin, as with all other histories, by introducing yourself, confirming the proposed surgery and her consent. You need to ask why she is having a shoulder replacement; is it for a fracture, OA, RA or some other reason. Then take a detailed past medical and surgical history.

2. Patients with RA presenting for joint replacement will tend to have relatively advanced disease. This may pose a number of problems as this disease can affect more than one body system. It is wise to ask about the following:
   - *Cardiovascular* – signs and symptoms of valvular disease, any previous echocardiography, diagnosis of past or current pericarditis, has she had a 12-lead ECG?
   - *Respiratory* – does she have any chest problems, is she ever short of breath and if so is there any suggestion of fibrosing alveolitis or pleural effusion?
   - *Joints* – which joints are most affected, what is her mobility like, does she have any spinal abnormalities or deformities (this will also have an impact on the respiratory system and ventilation)? Pay great attention to neck movements and think of the possibility of atlantoaxial subluxation. Positioning for surgery in these patients must be carefully planned
   - *Renal* – has she ever had vasculitis, does she have normal renal function (40 percent of patients with vasculitis have renal impairment)?
   - *Other* – does she have anemia, are there any clotting issues and, if she is on steroids, what is her skin quality like? Cannulation can be tricky and the skin may be prone to tearing, again having implications for moving and positioning while under anesthesia

3. There are many causes of chest pain and you will need to assess the type, severity and etiology. Broadly speaking, it could be cardiac, respiratory, gastric or musculoskeletal in origin. It will be useful to ask some of the following questions:
   - What type of pain is it, when does she get it, does it radiate, what makes it better, what makes it worse, does she get it at rest? It's important to determine if the pain may be cardiac ischemia (angina)
   - Is she hypertensive, has she had an MI in the past, is she known to have angina, are there any other strong cardiac risk factors?
   - Is the pain associated with exercise or deep breathing, does it hurt when she coughs, is she coughing up anything, like blood/sputum?
   - Does she take anything for the pain, does she use nitroglycerin, is she under the care of anyone, has she had it investigated – ECG, echo, chest X-ray, etc.?
   - Does she suffer with symptoms of reflux, could this simply be dyspepsia?

4. So far, you know that Mrs. Wood has RA and likely cardiac disease. You should be aware of the various cardiac drugs she is taking, in particular beta-blockers, calcium-channel antagonists and vasodilators. There are also a number of drugs used in the treatment of RA that are important:
   - *NSAIDs* – is she able to take nonsteroidals, does she take them currently? Be aware that if she has been on them long term, she may have a degree of renal impairment or gastric side effects
   - *Methotrexate* – this is a DMARD (disease modifying anti-rheumatoid drug) and may result in side effects such as nausea, mouth ulcers, skin thinning, pulmonary fibrosis,

altered liver function, aplastic anemia and pancytopenia. Be sure to look at a recent complete blood count (CBC) and clotting and liver function tests (LFTs)

- *Steroids* – usually low dose, but may be given in higher doses for a short period. Associated issues may be hyperglycemia, skin atrophy, and the need for intravenous steroid cover for long-term cases
- *Biologics* – these are monoclonal antibodies directed against tumor necrosis factor (TNFα) and increase the risk of infections, particularly tuberculosis. In some studies, but not all, they may also increase the risk of surgical site infections, lymphoma, and congestive heart failure

In addition, be aware of the potential issues surrounding patients that are immunosuppressed; for instance, risk of infection

5. Be sure to ask the anesthetic specific questions.
6. In such patients, you should prepare for a potentially difficult airway as a result of limited mouth opening and problems with neck movement. In addition to atlanto-occipital instability and cervical spine disease, they may also have temporomandibular and cricoarytenoid involvement.

   As mentioned previously, moving and positioning such a patient needs to be done extremely cautiously. Swollen and deformed joints can make peripheral access challenging. They can also give rise to pressure points, which are prone to breakdown. These patients are often frail in nature and need a gentle and carefully considered anesthetic. Regional techniques are favored by some in these cases, although they may be difficult to perform.
7. Given such information, you would want to perform a comprehensive airway assessment, look at the previous anesthetic chart, and consider the use of a fiber-optic scope or regional technique. It may be pertinent to get cervical spine imaging: X-ray, CT or MRI. You do not want to miss atlantoaxial subluxation or fractures of the odontoid process, risking a serious cervical spine injury during intubation.

5 Cesarean Section

Candidate's Instructions and Questions

Please take an appropriate history from Ms. King who is to have an elective cesarean section today.

How will you proceed and what are the important points to include in the history?

Answers

Generally speaking, young women coming for elective sections are healthy. The history taking therefore is centered on problems arising during pregnancy and why the woman is scheduled for a cesarean section. We will go through how to approach taking an obstetric history.

1. Introduction
   - Introduce yourself, check patient identity, confirm the consent and proposed procedure
2. Presenting history
   - Enquire as to the reason for having a cesarean section – previous sections, breech presentation, placenta previa/accreta, or traumatic labor the last time
   - Ask about problems during this pregnancy – urinary tract infections (UTIs), bleeding, anemia, syncope, abnormal scan results, high blood pressure, ankle swelling or proteinuria.
3. Past obstetric history
   - Any previous pregnancies/deliveries and any problems e.g. preeclampsia
   - Number of deliveries and mode of delivery, particularly cesarean section under spinal, epidural, or general anesthesia
   - What mode of analgesia did they use during previous labors, has the patient ever had an epidural and, if so, did it work for her?
4. Past medical and surgical history
   - Ask about any known medical problems
   - Ask about any previous surgery, in particular spinal surgery
   - Are there any current signs of infection or sepsis?
   - Include a detailed systems review as pregnancy impacts on almost every body system
   - Ask about cardiovascular problems, pre-existing hypertension, any history of valvular disease or cardiomyopathy
   - Has the patient any respiratory problems, asthma, recent upper or lower respiratory tract infections, is she able to lie flat?
   - If she has diabetes, how has it affected her pregnancy, is it well controlled, is it gestational, has she required insulin, are there any problems with the baby?
   - Has she suffered any musculoskeletal problems, back pain, sciatica, SPD (symphysis pubis dysfunction)? Record any sensory or motor dysfunction if present
   - Has the patient ever had any back surgery or particular spinal issues, spina bifida, intervertebral disc problems, fractures, etc? This is very important when considering regional anesthesia
   - Any clotting abnormalities or problems noted antenatally?
   - Try and assess venous access
5. Drug history
   - Allergies
   - Does the patient take any regular medication?
   - Women will usually be on folic acid and may be on iron supplements
   - Ask particularly if she has taken any ranitidine or other acid suppressants
6. Family history
   - Any family history of problems associated with anesthesia and, if so, what?
   - Is there a history of clotting disorders?

7. Anesthetic specific questions
   - Is the patient able to take nonsteroidal anti-inflammatory drugs (NSAIDs)?
   - Has she had previous general anesthetics, spinals or epidurals?
   - Does she smoke?
   - Note any problems with dentition
   - Ask about signs and symptoms of reflux – generally present in pregnant women
   - Assess neck movements and any musculoskeletal problems
   - Ask about weight and BMI; having a significantly raised BMI is increasingly common in this population and can make anesthetic management more challenging
   - Ask the patient if she has any particular concerns or questions

6 ENT Surgery

Candidate's Instructions and Questions

You are asked to take a history from a 27-year-old African-American who suffers with asthma and is presenting for ear, nose and throat (ENT) surgery.

1. How would you start your history?
2. What will you ask regarding his asthma?
3. Is there anything else, given the history, you want to know?

He tells you that he is having a tonsillectomy and was admitted with a severe asthma attack last year. He is not aware of any issues regarding sickle cell disease and he had surgery following a car accident some years ago.

4. What other questions might you ask?

He is having the tonsillectomy due to recurrent tonsillitis. He had his right leg pinned and arm plated after the accident; he no longer needs follow-up with the orthopedic surgeons. Drug history reveals that he takes long-term antibiotics.

5. Does the drug history concern you?

He plays rugby twice a week. He now remembers he also had a splenectomy following his car accident a few years ago.

6. What anesthetic specific questions will you ask?

Answers

1. Start your history by introducing yourself, checking the patient's identity and the consent form. You know he is having an ENT operation but you need to ascertain what the procedure is going to be as it is not specified in the instructions. Take a history of the presenting complaint and full past medical and surgical history. Even though the patient may appear young and healthy, there may be other factors involved.

2. You need to get a good respiratory history and should be asking questions such as:
   - How long has he had asthma, how does it affect his daily life, does he know his peak flow measurements, what is his exercise tolerance?
   - What medications does he take, is he compliant, how often does he take them, how often does he see his physician, how severe is his asthma?
   - Has he ever had any hospital admissions, when was his last asthma attack, is his asthma well controlled currently?
   - Does he have any signs of an upper or lower respiratory tract infection?

3. In this scenario the clue is that the patient is of African origin and it would be appropriate to ask about his sickle cell status. In an examination situation, you would be wise to ask about sickle cell disease and, indeed, thalassaemia. Its prevalence is high in people whose ancestors came from sub-Saharan Africa but extends, with lower prevalence, across the Arabian Peninsula into India.

   Anesthetic considerations are based around preventing a vaso-occlusive crisis, by ensuring adequate hydration, tissue oxygenation, normothermia and good analgesia. If the HbS level is high (> 30%), consider prophylactic blood transfusion.

4. He tells you he is having a tonsillectomy. This is a far more common procedure in children and it is important to know why an adult is having his tonsils removed. The reasons for adult tonsillectomy include:
   - Recurrent infections and tonsillitis
   - Peritonsillar abscess
   - Airway obstruction – performed for the same reason in adults as in children; tonsillar tissue overgrowth can obstruct the airway resulting in sleep apnea

   You need to ask details about his asthma attack and hospital admission. What were the events surrounding the admission, did he need ICU admission, was he intubated and ventilated and has he been followed up since. Again ask if he is compliant with medication and does he show any signs of current infection.

   Regarding the accident, you should ask exactly what surgeries he had, how long ago he had it, and did he have any problems or complications with the anesthetic?

5. A drug history can sometimes highlight things that a patient may not have told you about in his/her past medical or surgical history. Ask why he is on long-term antibiotic therapy. Some reasons include:
   - Bronchiectasis, recurrent urinary tract infections, organ transplants, post-splenectomy, acne, and experimentally (off label) for lupus or Crohn's disease

   In this scenario, his splenectomy has resulted in the need for long-term antibiotics. You could also ask if the patient received the recommended vaccines.

6. By now, you should know to always ask:
   - Any previous anesthetics, including family history of any problems?
   - Any issues with dentition?

- Any symptoms of acid reflux or indigestion?
- Any neck problems?
- Has he met the NPO policy?
- Is he taking nonsteroidal anti-inflammatory drugs (NSAIDs)?
- Smoking, drug, and alcohol history

Introduction

The vast array of clinical situations in which you can find yourself makes preparation for the communication stations rather difficult. These scenarios are designed to test candidates on a number of levels:

- Clinical acumen
- Anesthetic knowledge
- Ability to break bad news
- Situational awareness
- Issues regarding capacity and consent
- Personal characteristics of compassion and empathy

In the communication stations, there will be a number of issues that the patient will want to address. In contrast to the history-taking stations where the candidate takes the lead, the patient will be asking you the questions. On occasion, the patient may become upset or angry; for example, if you have to talk to a relative about the death of a family member. Be prepared for this, try to remain calm and do not get flustered. You are likely to have dealt with similar situations in real life so draw on your previous experiences. Communication stations are likely to fall into one of three categories:

1. Practical procedures

   - Explain a rapid sequence induction (RSI) to a patient
   - Talk about and explain epidural analgesia to a patient undergoing an esophagogastrectomy
   - Order blood over the phone during a postpartum hemorrhage
   - Hand over a patient to a member of recovery staff

2. Counselling

   - Talk to a patient with a post-dural puncture headache
   - Discuss analgesia with an intravenous drug user
   - Discuss blood transfusion with a Jehovah's Witness
   - Explain the anesthetic implications of a heart murmur

3. Breaking bad news

   - Tell someone his/her relative has been admitted to the intensive care unit
   - Talk to a patient with nerve damage following spinal anesthesia
   - Talk to patient who suffered anaphylaxis due to a drug error

To go through all possible communication scenarios is beyond the scope of this book but this chapter will run through six communication stations, mainly based on the authors' experiences. There are suggested candidate responses coupled with potential patient questions and remarks.

1 Sickle Cell Test

Candidate's Instructions

You are asked to preoperatively assess an Afro–Caribbean patient who is having elective surgery. He is unsure of his sickle cell status. You want to take a blood sample and perform a sickle cell test. Please explain this to the patient and obtain his consent for the blood test.

This station will not be as straightforward as simply obtaining consent for a blood test. There is likely to be another underlying issue and it is important that you tease this out of the patient and address the problem to gain full points. Start by introducing yourself and obtain a more detailed history from the patient:

- Confirm that he is to undergo surgery and ask what the operation is
- Ask again about his sickle cell status
- Ask about any family history of sickle cell disease

Continue by explaining why it is important to know a patient's sickle cell status prior to any operation and outline some reasons why.

- It may determine the mode of anesthesia used; for instance, regional over general anesthesia
- You may need to discuss his status with the hematologists preoperatively
- There are risks of proceeding without knowing his sickle cell status

Inform him that it is routine for certain patient groups to be tested for sickle cell disease. Explain that it will be a quick blood test that should take less than a minute and that he will be tested for sickle cell disease only and nothing else will be tested for without his consent. Obtain consent for the blood test.

He Is Not Enthusiastic and Refuses to Have the Blood Test

You will then need to ask about his specific concerns regarding the test and why he does not want it done. Address any issues he may have and be sympathetic to his needs.

When Asked, It Transpires that He Is Needle Phobic

Stress the importance of having the test done and why you need to know his sickle cell status.

- It may harm him if you proceed without knowing
- Special attention may need to be given to fluid management, analgesia and oxygenation if he tests positive
- It may have implications for his future health

Then run through some options for venipuncture in the needle-phobic patient:

- You can offer local anesthetic cream
- Offer to draw the blood test yourself
- Explain you will take your time to find the best site for venipuncture

- Say you will use the smallest needle possible
- Offer distraction techniques or the presence of a family member
- Reassure him that it will be quick and as painless as possible

Eventually He Agrees to Have the Test Done

End the station by thanking the patient for his cooperation and summarize your agreed plan of action.

2 Rapid Sequence Induction

Candidate's Instructions

You are asked to explain an RSI to a 32-year-old woman who is on the emergency schedule for an appendectomy. She has a fear of masks and does not want preoxygenation.

Begin by introducing yourself and confirming that the patient is to have the proposed operation. Try and make the patient feel comfortable and aim to establish a good rapport in the first few minutes. If you know she has a phobia of masks, it may be best to address this last. Explain the nature of an RSI and why we use it.

- It is a type of anesthetic that we use for emergency surgery
- Discuss the operating room and establishing intravenous access, an ECG, blood pressure cuff and pulse oximetry
- Make her aware that there will be two or three people present in the operating room to help you and put her at ease
- Talk about cricoid pressure. Explain that it will be done just as she is going off to sleep and that it is important to prevent any stomach contents coming up the wrong way and into the lungs
- Then discuss preoxygenation, approach the subject carefully, asking about her concerns and previous experiences

    At this point, the patient becomes anxious and says she will not have the mask anywhere near her.

    Explore the reasons why she has a fear of masks, was it a previous anesthetic? If so, for what, where and when?

    Explain the importance of preoxygenation in this setting; for example:

- It is needed to help fill your lungs with as much oxygen as possible
- It provides a large reservoir of oxygen during the start of the anesthetic and is required to help make the induction of anesthesia as safe as possible
- We will continuously monitor your oxygen levels using a probe placed on your finger

    Discuss the various options available for preoxygenation.

- She can hold the mask herself, although a close seal is required
- Offer her a facemask to familiarize herself with beforehand
- She can take three to five maximum inspiratory breaths before induction as opposed to a three-minute tidal volume preoxygenation
- Explain the masks are clear and feel less claustrophobic than the black masks some people remember
- Tell her there will be a number of people present to look after her
- Reassure her that it is routine and you will be there to look after her
- Explore the possibility of a nasal cannula pre- and postoperatively

3 Succinylcholine Apnea

Candidate's Instructions

Mr. Dale's 6-year-old daughter has just undergone emergency surgery and currently is being ventilated in the intensive care unit (ICU). It is thought she has pseudocholinesterase deficiency. You are asked to talk to him and explain what has happened.

In this situation, be acutely aware that the parent is likely to be very anxious and upset and may not have any understanding as to what has happened. Introduce yourself, be calm and comforting.

Ask what the father already knows.

- How much does he understand about the situation so far?
- Expand on what he knows and give a brief summary of the events
- Allow him to ask any questions he may have and respond to them sympathetically
- Provide factual, structured answers. Do not beat about the bush

There are a number of issues you should address here.

What Has Happened and What Is Pseudocholinesterase Deficiency?

- In order for your daughter to have her surgery, we used a drug called succinylcholine as part of the anesthetic. It is routinely used for emergency surgery to relax the muscles
- Sometimes the drug takes longer than expected to wear off and stop working. It is a recognized but rare complication of using succinylcholine
- Consequently, we are keeping her asleep in the ICU while closely monitoring her muscle power. Once her muscles have regained their full strength, we will wake her up
- There will be no long-term effects
- This problem occurs as a result of different enzymes produced by a gene and is an inherited condition
- Because her muscles, including those she uses for breathing, are not yet working as they should, she is not able to breathe fully
- It can take a number of hours to wear off and for her to breathe normally

Be reassuring and allow time for the information to sink in. Let the father ask any questions as you go along.

What Is the Current Situation and Will She Breathe Again?

- Currently, a breathing machine known as a ventilator is assisting her breathing
- She is being kept asleep while it assists her breathing and she will not be in pain or discomfort. It is a bit like a long anesthetic

- We are monitoring her muscle movement and when she starts to breathe for herself we will wake her up and take her off the ventilator
- She will then breathe as she would normally

What Will Happen after This?

- This episode is not likely to affect your daughter's recovery following her surgery
- However, pseudocholinesterase deficiency can be a result of genetic variations and can be inherited. It is advisable that your daughter and direct family members be referred for testing and we will make the arrangements for you
- Your daughter will be issued with a warning card and succinylcholine should be avoided in the future

These suggested questions are examples of some that may arise or ones you may want to cover in your explanation to the father.

Obviously, the order in which you explain things may be dictated by the actor. Take on board the parent's requests and honor them where possible.

4 Cancelled Surgery

Candidate's Instructions

Mr. Young has had his elective hernia repair cancelled as there was an emergency laparotomy. You are asked to go and see him and tell him the news as the surgeon and his team are busy in the operating room.

This is really a breaking bad news scenario. Prepare and compose yourself during the time before starting the station as the patient is likely to be angry and confrontational. Take a moment to think about how you will explain the situation; be sympathetic but as direct and factual as possible.

A suggested way to approach this station is:

- Introduce yourself fully, confirm the patient's identity and inform him that you are the anesthesiologist
- Find out what he knows so far; that is, has anybody told him you were coming to see him? Have the nursing staff told him anything?
- Approach the matter calmly and say; for example, "Unfortunately, things have not quite gone as planned this morning" and wait for his response
- Explain that there has been an emergency procedure that needed to be done and, therefore, his operation has been cancelled. Be assertive but sympathetic
- Apologize for the inconvenience and reiterate that the laparotomy was life-saving surgery. Indicate that by giving up his slot he has helped someone who was seriously unwell
- Try and empathize with him; he is likely to be hungry and thirsty and to have been awake since early morning
- Tell him that you will speak with his surgeon and the surgeon will reschedule him
- Tell him the surgeon will also come and talk to him
- Make sure he understands that his surgery will not be today
- Again apologize and ask him if he has any questions

The patient may respond by asking to be put on the afternoon schedule. Reiterate that that will be up to his surgeon.

If the patient wishes to take things further, do not try to dissuade him. Be understanding of his situation and inform him that he can write or call the patient representative or ombudsman at the hospital.

5 Dental Damage

Candidate's Instructions

While intubating Mr. Davies, you knock out one of his front teeth. You failed preoperatively to mention tooth damage as a potential risk. It is now a few hours since the operation and you go to his room to explain what has happened.

The patient is going to be upset and angry at the loss of his tooth so prepare yourself and try not to get flustered if he becomes confrontational and aggressive. A proposed way of approaching this situation is as follows:

- If possible, indicate that you would like to have a member of the nursing staff present as a witness during the conversation with Mr. Davies
- Introduce yourself briefly, he is likely to remember who you are and may pass comment to such effect
- Be extremely apologetic at all times and speak calmly and sympathetically
- Explain that there was a problem getting the endotracheal tube in and that, unfortunately, you caught one of his teeth in doing so. Do not make it sound as though you are blaming him and make sure he understands that you accept responsibility for the event
- If he asks why you did not tell him about tooth damage before the surgery, it is best to admit that you failed to mention it and say you are sorry rather than go down other routes
- You will need to explain what will happen next and tell him that you will do everything possible to help amend the situation as quickly and effectively as possible
- Ask if he has any pain or discomfort and offer appropriate analgesia if required
- Say you will personally arrange an appointment with a dentist as a matter of urgency
- If he wishes to visit his own dentist, inform him you will contact his dentist explaining the situation and try and expedite the appointment
- Many anesthesiology groups will usually cover reasonable costs for dental injury as a matter of business expenses and the desire to avoid a malpractice suit. If the tooth was rotted and hanging only by a thread, anesthesiologists usually don't offer to financially cover but if it was a solid tooth most will pay
- Again apologize and reassure him that you will do your very best to help him with further management
- Tell him that you have discussed this case with risk management and ask him if he would like to speak with them about the events
- If he wishes to take the matter further in terms of a hospital complaint, do not try and dissuade him. Offer him the patient representative or ombudsman
- Say you will write to his primary care physician and dentist explaining what has happened
- End apologetically and ask Mr. Davies if he has any questions or if there is anything more you could do for him

6 Jehovah's Witness

Candidate's Instructions

You are asked to see Mrs. Smart in the antenatal clinic. She is 34 weeks pregnant and due to have an elective cesarean section in four weeks' time. She is a Jehovah's Witness with a current hemoglobin of 9.2 g/dL. Please obtain her consent for cesarean section without the use of blood products.

The important issues to address are:

- What blood products and methods of transfusion are acceptable to the patient
- Risks of refusing blood transfusion
- Current anemia and treatment thereof
- Anesthetic techniques
- Multidisciplinary approach to her care
- There may be a specific consent form for Jehovah's Witness and other patients who decline blood products

Start by introducing yourself and confirming the proposed procedure. Confirm that Mrs. Smart is a Jehovah's Witness and explore her exact beliefs further. It is important to know what blood products she will and will not accept.

- Jehovah's Witnesses will **not accept** whole blood, fresh frozen plasma, platelets, packed red cells or autologous predonation but be sure to check, particularly regarding the latter
- Products that **may be acceptable** to use include albumin, and clotting factors, such as prothrombin complex and activated factor seven
- In this case, you must ask in particular about **cell salvage** and whether or not the patient will consent to its use. Some Jehovah's Witnesses will only consent to its use if there is a continuous circuit between machine and body, so check!
- Ask about the acceptability of erythropoietin and intravenous iron
- Establish whether or not she has an "Advanced Directive" and ask exactly what it states

You will need to explain fully the risks of not accepting blood products in the event of excessive blood loss; that is, the increased risk of hysterectomy, admission to ICU and, potentially, death.

Ensure that she appreciates how serious it may be but try not to be confrontational: "Just to confirm, am I right in saying that even if a blood transfusion could prevent your death you would refuse the transfusion?"

Address the issue of anemia at the present time and say that it would be wise to optimize her hemoglobin before surgery.

- Suggest that she takes ferrous sulfate preoperatively
- Explain that you will discuss further management of her anemia with a hematologist as she may benefit from recombinant erythropoietin if she is willing to take it

If the patient asks about anesthetic management of her surgery, it would be sensible to mention the following:

- Involvement of an anesthesiologist and an obstetrician
- Regional technique preferred to general anesthesia
- Meticulous hemostasis and avoidance of hypothermia
- Potential use of invasive monitoring and its benefits
- The use of a cell saver if the patient consents

You will also write to her obstetrician indicating what you have discussed and any management you have implemented.

If not done so already, make sure that the Mrs. Smart has signed the consent form used for patients who decline blood transfusions.

Ask Mrs. Smart if she has any further questions. Summarize briefly what she is willing to accept and make sure this has been documented.

1 Electrocautery

Electrocautery was first used in Spain in the early 1900s and advances in modern machines have revolutionized surgery today. It is commonplace in the operating rooms and, as anesthesiologists, you need to know enough about it to help out your surgical colleagues or protect your patient. Therefore, if the questions seem to be leading towards electro-cautery, think alternating current (AC) and direct current (DC), frequency, capacitance, and safety features.

Questions

1. What is meant by electrocautery and what modes are there?
2. How does electrocautery cause coagulation?
3. What potential dangers are there?
4. Can electrocautery be used on patients with pacemakers?
5. What is capacitive coupling?

Answers

1. Electrocautery describes a device that uses the heat generated by an electrical current to cauterize, cut or ablate tissue. It is commonly used as unipolar or bipolar.

2. The key here is **current density**. The higher the current density, the greater the amount of heat energy present. Unipolar devices consist of an electrode at the surgical end and a ground plate attached to the patient. Electrical current passes from the electrocautery tip to this plate. The current density is highest at the tip as it has a much smaller diameter and surface area than the ground plate. The heat produced at the cautery tip causes cauterization and hence hemostasis. Note that the current used for electrocautery is of very high frequency at around 500,000 to 1,000,000 Hz.

   Bipolar devices do not require a neutral plate as the electrosurgical current flows between the forceps tips.

3. Cautery is used in many surgical procedures. You should have an understanding of how it works and the dangers involved with its use. They include:

   - Thermal burns to the patient if the ground plate is not smoothly and completely adherent to the skin
   - If unipolar electrocautery is used on an area raised on a pedicle (e.g. the testicle on the spermatic cord), then the pedicle will be the only route for current to pass and will become the region of highest current density, thus producing burns
   - Electrocautery may ignite inflammable media such as an alcohol-based skin preparation
   - Electrocautery can also cause electrical interference with other devices such as ECG monitors

4 & 5. Yes, but it should be used only when absolutely necessary and, even then, preferentially used as bipolar, as the electrosurgical current is localized to the forceps tips. There is the risk of damage to the pacemaker or accidental inhibition of function. The pacemaker has conducting materials in direct contact with the heart and burns are possible at these sites. Microshock is also a cause for concern. If electrical current passes through the device, capacitive coupling is a natural occurrence that can happen when energy is transferred through intact insulating materials to a conductor. It refers to the transfer of energy to different devices that are linked via an electrical network. This can present a problem during laparoscopic procedures where the cautery electrode is activated when not in direct contact with tissues. This turns the patient into one plate of a capacitor, the probe being the other plate and the carbon dioxide in the pneumoperitoneum functioning as the capacitor dielectric. In an AC system, potentially operating at 1 MHz, this can cause burns distant from the electrocautery site.

Discussion

The physical principles of cautery are straightforward and, therefore, this could be a potentially easy station, requiring a small amount of preparation. You may well have heard the surgeon talk about switching the electrocautery from "coagulation" to "cutting," and it is important to know that this refers to the waveform of the electrocautery current rather than the mode; all the waveforms can be utilized in each mode. The waveform for cutting is a sine wave and for coagulation a damped, intermittent waveform is best. Blend (or "spray") is a shorter wavelength, with a damped sine waveform.

2 Defibrillators

Hot on the heels of electrocautery comes every examiner's favorite capacitance question. Perhaps more likely in the written examination than in the OSCE, but this could certainly occur as part of a question on resuscitation or a lead-on from electrocautery.

Questions

1. What types of defibrillator are there?
2. How do external defibrillators work?
3. What are the advantages of biphasic defibrillators?
4. Look at this defibrillator circuit diagram and name the components labelled A, B and C.

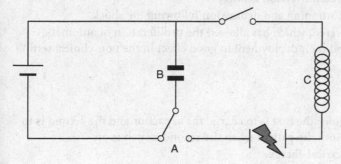

5. What do A, B and C do?

Answers

1. Defibrillators can be divided broadly into external defibrillators and internal defibrillators (implanted cardioverting defibrillators [ICDs]). External defibrillators can be further subdivided into monophasic or biphasic, based on the waveform produced.
2. Defibrillators are designed to provide a quantity of electrical energy in the form of direct current (DC) to the myocardium in order to return normal rhythm to a fibrillating heart. The energy required is set on the control panel; this energy is then stored in a capacitor and discharged into the patient via two large electrode pads (or paddles) placed across the chest wall or the chest and back. Although it is not fully understood, it is thought that the energy wave causes prolongation of the refractory period of the heart muscle, which will allow aberrant depolarization to fade away and normal rhythm to resume.
3. Biphasic defibrillators reverse the polarity of the shock midway through shock delivery. Advantages include:
   - The energy required for cardioversion is lower
   - There is less myocardial stunning and depression following the shock
   - They can be battery powered, which has allowed the proliferation of automatic external defibrillators and their deployment to good effect in the non-clinical setting
4. A: Switch
   B: Capacitor
   C: Inductor
5. A: Switch A has two functions: the first is to charge the capacitor and the second is to discharge the capacitor into the patient when the second switch is on
   B: The capacitor stores electrical charge
   C: The inductor causes a back electromotive force to deliberately slow down the discharge rate of the defibrillator as this leads to improved chance of success

Discussion

The charge and energy stored by a capacitor are described by:

Charge (coulombs) = Capacitance (farads) × Voltage (volts)
$Q = C \times V$
Energy (joules) $= \frac{1}{2}CV^2$

Defibrillators use a step-up transformer to convert 120 V alternating current (AC) into 5,000 V DC. The standard energy used for defibrillation is:
- Monophasic: 360 J
- Biphasic: 150 J
- ICD: 30–50 J

ICDs are fitted like a pacemaker and an ever-growing proportion of the population has them. Speaking with the patient's ICD service prior to anesthesia is strongly recommended and the usual pacemaker precautions should be employed.

3 Laryngoscopes

This is a large topic and the questions could go in many directions. There are a multitude of laryngoscopes available and you are highly unlikely to have used most of them. It could also touch on the anatomy of the upper airway and pharmacology of local anesthetics.

Questions

1. Look at the following pictures and name the different laryngoscopes.

(a)

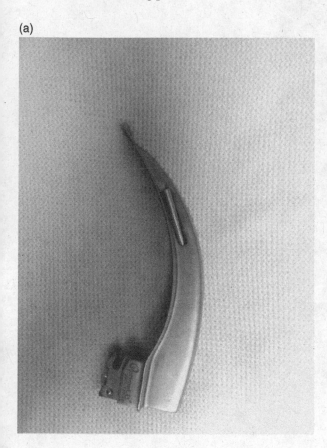

(b)

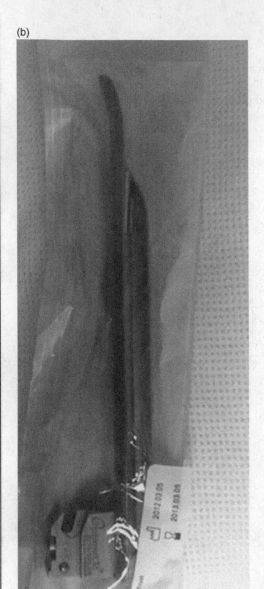

(c)

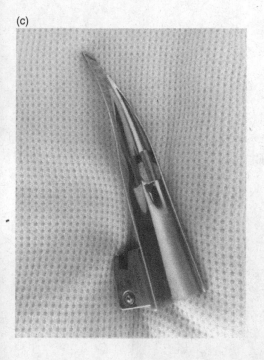

(d)

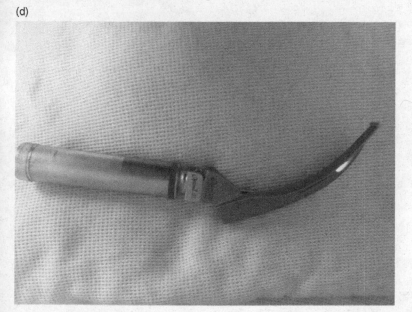

(e)

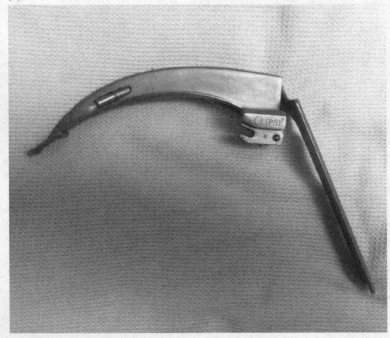

(f)

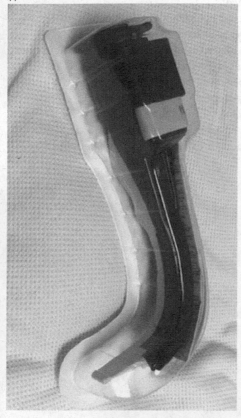

(g)

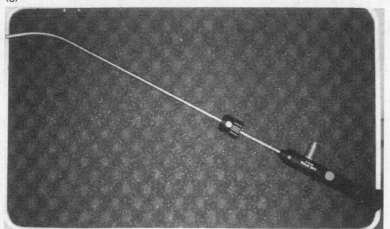

2. What are the features of a Macintosh laryngoscope blade?
3. How should reusable laryngoscopes be cleaned?
4. Why are there straight and curved laryngoscope blades?
5. Outline the Cormack and Lehane grades of view at laryngoscopy.
6. What is the difference between a traditional Macintosh laryngoscope and a rigid fiber-optic laryngoscope such as the Glidescope or McGrath video laryngoscope?
7. There are a large number of different rigid fiber-optic laryngoscopes available. Why have these not replaced flexible fiber-optic laryngoscopes?
8. A patient presents for an emergency laparotomy, and tells you that due to previous radiotherapy he/she has very limited mouth opening (approximately 1.5 cm) and poor neck movement. Outline a reasonable technique for intubation of this patient.

Answers

1. A: Macintosh
   B: Miller
   C: Robertshaw
   D: Polio
   E: McCoy
   F: AirTraq
   G: Bonfils

2. A handle with detachable blade. The handle contains a battery; the blade contains either a bulb mounted on the end or a fiber-optic bundle that transmits light from a bulb located in the handle. The blade is available in a variety of sizes (1–4) and also in disposable formats.

3. Traditionally, just soap and water was used; however, most hospitals now sterilize laryngoscope blades after each use. Methods of sterilization include ethylene oxide, autoclave or gamma irradiation. The handle must be cleaned as well: specialized anti-microbial wipes must be used.

4. Straight blades are designed to be used in a different way to curved blades. With a curved blade, one aims the tip into the vallecula and the bulbous tip lifts the epiglottis by traction on ligaments, the laryngoscope can be inserted in the midline and the blade has a section designed to retract the tongue out of the way. Straight blades are designed to lift the epiglottis out of the way. Narrow profile blades like the Miller laryngoscope are not as effective in the midline as they cannot retract the tongue.

5. The Cormack and Lehane system for grading laryngoscopy is as follows:

Grade I	All of glottis visible
Grade II	Portion of anterior glottis not visible
Grade III	Only epiglottis visible
Grade IV	Epiglottis not visible

6. The principle difference is that with the traditional Macintosh blade, one is aiming to retract the tissues of the mouth until a line of sight from the anesthesiologist to the patient's glottis is formed. Rigid fiber-optic laryngoscopes transmit the image of the glottis to a screen or eye-piece, allowing the anesthesiologist to "see round corners," potentially turning a poor laryngoscopic view into a good one. In order to enhance the view obtained, most of these laryngoscopes have a more pronounced blade curvature than the Macintosh blade.

7. Most of the rigid fiber-optic laryngoscopes are bulky and are not suitable for patients with extremely limited or no mouth opening. For these, nasal intubation using a flexible fiber-optic scope may be the best option. Lack of familiarity and limited evidence surrounding the efficacy and safety profiles of the newer rigid fiber-optic laryngoscopes also contribute to their restricted use. This may well change in the near future.

8. Awake fiber-optic nasal intubation is the best technique here as the patient is likely to be at significant risk of aspiration and has very limited mouth opening. The patient must be cooperative and have the procedure fully explained to him/her. Adequate local

anesthesia of the upper airway can be achieved with a variety of techniques: topical spray of local anesthetic or superior laryngeal nerve blocks. A vasoconstrictor can be sprayed into the nose with local anesthetic (e.g. oxymetazoline or phenylephrine). An anti-sialagog (e.g. glycopyrrolate 200 µg IV) is recommended. A flexible fiber-optic laryngo-scope with an appropriate endotracheal tube (ETT) preloaded can then be used to intubate the patient. General anesthesia can commence once correct endotracheal placement is confirmed. A full description of awake fiber-optic intubation is beyond the scope of this book.

Discussion

- There are a large number of laryngoscopes available: no one type is perfect for every patient
- Macintosh did not design the pediatric sizes of his blade: in fact, he condemned them as being the wrong shape for the pediatric airway
- Sterilization of laryngoscope blades causes ongoing damage, especially to fiber-optic light bundles, and reduces brightness and hence effectiveness
- There have been case reports of cross-infection where the laryngoscope handle had not been cleaned properly between uses
- A straight blade technique is not taught often with the advent of fiber-optic laryngoscopes; however, it is worth watching an ear, nose and throat (ENT) surgeon insert the straight, rigid, operating laryngoscope to appreciate the technique. A better view may be possible with a straight blade than you were able to obtain with a curved blade. Both techniques are worth learning
- Rigid fiber-optic laryngoscopes, turning a grade IV view into a grade I view, are extremely useful but it does not always follow that it becomes an easy intubation as the ETT must be manipulated "round the corner." The other problem with rigid fiber-optic laryngoscopes is that the window transmitting the image from the distal tip of the blade is often small and, therefore, easily obscured by blood or secretions
- It is always worth remembering older techniques: blind nasal intubation in the spontaneously breathing patient with no mouth opening was used prior to flexible fiber-optic laryngoscopy
- Awake fiber-optic intubation: it is important not to forget extubation. A significant number of airway disasters occur at extubation. The patient described earlier is still at risk of aspiration postoperatively; therefore, an appropriate plan for extubation must be made (including the fact that emergency re-intubation will not be easy). Decompress the stomach using a nasogastric tube and treat the patient with agents to reduce gastric acid.

4 Endotracheal Tubes

In anesthesia, it is common to hear people talking about "tubing," rather than intubating, "tubed" and so on. Please fight against it! Treat the examination as a time for blossoming professionalism, try and avoid a casual style and adopt a professional, formal manner. This station will be your real test. Knowledge of the various types and uses of endotracheal tubes (ETTs) will be essential.

Questions

1. Look at picture A. What is it? List the design features.

(a)

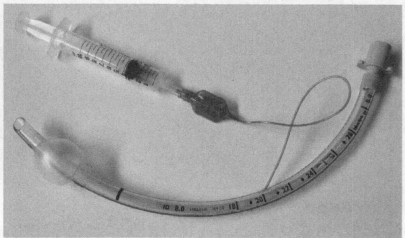

2. Explain the different types of cuffs found on ETTs and the rationale for each type.
3. When are uncuffed tubes used?
4. What are the hazards of endotracheal intubation?
5. What is an endobronchial blocker? How is it placed?
6. What is the alternative to an endobronchial blocker?

7. Look at the following pictures. Name these different tubes and what they are used for.

(b)

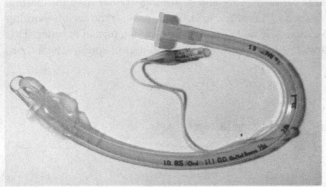

(c)

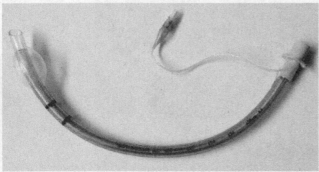

(d)

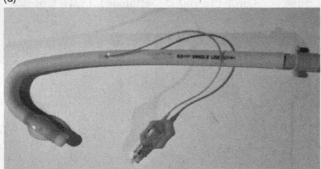

(e)

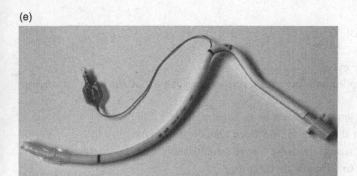

8.   How does jet ventilation work? When is it contraindicated?
9.   Outline the differences between a percutaneous and surgical tracheostomy.

Answers

1. A cuffed, oral ETT, size 8.0.
   Features:
   - Bevel tip with Murphy eye
   - A cuff connected to a pilot balloon with a self-closing valve that allows inflation and deflation of the cuff
   - Markings to show the length of the tube in centimeters
   - Markings to show that the material has been tested for toxicity
   - Markings to show the size of the tube (its internal diameter in millimeters)
   - A connector to attach to a breathing circuit

2. *High-volume, low-pressure cuffs*: for longer-term intubation; for example, in an intensive-care setting, the cuff has a large surface area of contact with the tracheal wall to help prevent tissue damage and necrosis.
   Low-volume, high-pressure cuffs: for short-term use where a tight seal is needed to prevent tracheal soiling. These are rarely used anymore.
   Double cuffs: for example, on laser tubes, in case one cuff ruptures.

3. Uncuffed tubes are more commonly used in pediatric anesthesia. The narrowest part of the pediatric airway is at the level of the cricoid cartilage.

4. The main risks of endotracheal intubation are:
   - Tooth damage
   - Injury to soft tissues including the lips and arytenoids
   - Tracheal wall damage and tracheal perforation (very rare)
   - Postoperative sore throat and uvula swelling
   - Misplacement of the tube
   - Delayed recognition of esophageal intubation

5. This is a long, thin tube with a cuff that is passed through a normal ETT beyond the carina into either the left or right main bronchus and then inflated so as to isolate a lung for surgery requiring access to a hemithorax. It is placed using a fiber-optic broncho-scope with the bronchial blocker preloaded onto the scope so that it can be placed under direct vision.

6. Double lumen tubes (DLTs) with tracheal and bronchial tubes and cuffs are more commonly used. DLTs are specifically right- or left-sided tubes. Right-sided tubes have a bronchial tube-and-cuff that sits in the right main bronchus, whereas left-sided tubes have a bronchial tube-and-cuff that is placed into the left main bronchus. Commonly, a left-sided DLT is used as this avoids the risk of occluding the right upper bronchus when placing a right-sided DLT. Examples of DLTs are the Bronchocath, the Robertshaw tube and the Carlen's tube, which has a carinal hook to aid placement.

7. B: South-facing Ring–Adair–Elwyn (RAE) tube: used so that the external component of the tube is out of the surgical field in ENT and oral surgery.
   C: Flexometallic or armored tube: designed to prevent kinking or compression of the tube; useful in surgery where the airway may be inaccessible (e.g. in the prone position) or for when massive airway edema may complicate the future course of the patient.

D: Montandon tube: to replace a tracheostomy for ongoing surgical procedures where the bulk of a tracheostomy tube would be in the surgeon's way.

E: Portex Ivory nasal tube: soft material designed to minimize trauma to the nasal passages.

8. Jet ventilation can be achieved either via a dedicated jet catheter using high-frequency jet ventilation, or via a transtracheal catheter or intravenous cannula in an emergency, or via a channel on a rigid bronchoscope using the ManuJet or Sanders injector. Manual jet ventilation uses high-flow oxygen delivered for brief periods of time through an appropriate airway; air is entrained by the Venturi effect. Barotrauma and pneumothorax are possible. Crucially, expiration is passive so a patent upper airway is required in order to prevent gas trapping and cardiovascular collapse.

9. A percutaneous tracheostomy uses a tracheal dilator over a guidewire inserted by percutaneous needle puncture of the trachea to create the tracheal stoma. A surgical tracheostomy requires dissection of the overlying structures, direct visualization of the trachea and formation of a stoma.

Discussion

- The Murphy eye is designed to allow ventilation even if the open end of the tube is blocked by secretions or occluded by the tracheal wall
- Nitrous oxide can diffuse into endotracheal cuffs and increase the pressure, potentially causing pressure-related tissue ischemia or necrosis of the trachea. There are various tubes available that are designed to overcome this with cuff pressure monitoring
- RAE stands for Ring–Adair–Elwyn who were Canadian anesthesiologists who developed the tube
- Bronchial blockers are tricky to insert and are associated with a relatively high failure rate. There is a new endotracheal tube, the Papworth Bivent tube, designed to facilitate placement of an endobronchial blocker. The bivent tube is a straight DLT with no endobronchial arm. Instead, it is passed down to sit on the carina and each side has a hole designed to face the respective main bronchus. Thus, an endobronchial blocker can be placed through either the right- or left-hand side and be guided into place more easily. The Rusch® EZ-blocker is another form of bronchial blocker placed down a single lumen tube. It has two cuffs and also sits on the carina, allowing either cuff to be inflated

5 Breathing Circuits

There will almost certainly be a question on breathing systems and part of it will likely be to check a circuit.

Questions

1. What is the name of this circuit? What is its Mapleson classification?

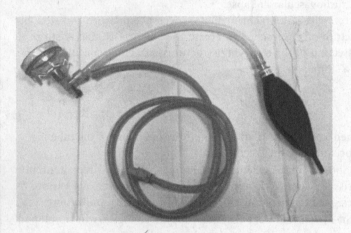

2. This circuit is attached to an anesthetic machine at the common gas outlet. Check that the circuit is safe to use.
3. You discover a tear in the bag: if you had not discovered that tear, what problems could this generate during anesthesia?
4. What could you do to eliminate this problem?
5. Name two components commonly attached to all circuits that are not on this one.
6. What is the volume of the bag? What is the volume of the reservoir tubing?
7. What group of patients is this circuit used for? Up to what weight?
8. Name two advantages of using it in this population.
9. Name two disadvantages.
10. What modifications could eliminate these disadvantages?
11. What is the minimum fresh gas flow rate required for a spontaneously ventilating patient to prevent rebreathing?
12. How does one perform intermittent positive pressure ventilation (IPPV) with this circuit?
13. How can positive end-expiratory pressure (PEEP) be applied for the spontaneously breathing patient?
14. Which Mapleson system is most efficient for spontaneously breathing patients and which for ventilated patients?

Answers

1. This is a Jackson–Rees modification of Ayre's T-Piece (Mapleson F classification). (Ayre's T-Piece was the same without the open-ended reservoir bag.)
   Mapleson classified breathing systems into A, B, C, D and E. After further revision of the classification, the F breathing system was added.

2. State that you would do a machine check first but there is not time to do both in the examination so the examiners will tell you that it has been checked and is safe.
   For the circuit check, follow a well-practiced logical routine:
   - Check all tubing is patent
   - Check for foreign bodies in any part of it (that is why all tubing/connectors must now be semi-transparent)
   - Check the bag tail is patent
   - Fill the circuit with oxygen, occlude the patient connection and bag tail to check that it can be pressurized and examine for any holes/tears/leaks

3. You would be unable to pressurize the bag, therefore unable to establish IPPV, and gas escaping during spontaneous breathing would necessitate higher fresh gas flows.

4. If the patient is spontaneously ventilating, turn the fresh gas flow up and seek a replacement bag. If you are manually ventilating the patient, remove the bag and attach the reservoir tubing to a ventilator.

5. Two commonly found components are:
   - Heat and moisture exchange filter between mask and circuit
   - Sample line for gas monitoring and capnography (mainstream/sidestream)

6. The volume of the bag is 500 mL. The tubing volume depends on length (about 200 mL normally)

7. A Mapleson F is commonly used for pediatric anesthesia in children up to a weight of 30 kg. (**Note:** some books say up to 20 kg; most pediatric anesthesiologists are happy to use up to 30 kg and beyond, in some cases.)

8. Advantages include: lightweight, low dead space, low resistance to expiration and inexpensive.

9. Disadvantages include: no scavenging, no adjustable pressure limiting (APL) valve and high fresh gas flows are required to prevent rebreathing.

10. The addition of an APL valve and closed reservoir bag allows scavenging.

11. Minimum fresh gas flow of 2.5–3 times the minute ventilation is required to prevent rebreathing.

12. To ventilate manually using a Mapleson F, partially occlude the reservoir bag tail and hand ventilate or remove the bag and plug onto a ventilator.

13. PEEP can be applied by partially occluding the reservoir bag while the patient is spontaneously breathing.

14. For spontaneously ventilating patients, the order of efficiency for the Mapleson breathing systems is A > DEF > BC.
    For controlled ventilation, the order of efficiency is DFE > BC > A.

Discussion

- Go through these questions for each of the Mapleson breathing circuits. There are a lot of common elements
- Learn the fresh gas flow requirements for each circuit for both spontaneous and controlled ventilation
- Mapleson A and D circuits come as co-axial systems as well. Adaptation into co-axial systems produces specific advantages for each system but also specific disadvantages: think of APL valve position/weight on the endotracheal tube and how to test for patency and leaks

6 Airways

Dr. Archie Brain, an Oxford scholar, patented the laryngeal mask airway (LMA) in 1982 and drastically changed the face of modern anesthesia. If the LMA comes up in a station, it is likely that the examiner will focus on the applications, design features and safe usage of these devices.

Questions

1. What are the components of an anesthetic facemask?
2. What airway adjuncts are available?
3. What are the indications for using an LMA?
4. What are the contraindications?
5. What are the "second generation" supraglottic airway devices?

Answers

1. The *mount*: a 22-mm female taper.
   The *body*: this should be rigid enough to hold against the face without distorting the mask.
   The *edge*: this is usually an inflatable cuff to provide a gas-tight seal. Virtually all hospitals now use single patient-use facemasks.
2. Oropharyngeal or nasopharyngeal airways. The oropharyngeal or Guedel airway comes in a variety of sizes for all ages, as do nasopharyngeal airways.
3. Indications:
   - Primarily designed to replace a facemask anesthetic
   - Short procedures for patients who are spontaneously breathing
   - Emergency use in a "cannot intubate, cannot ventilate" scenario
   - To provide a smooth emergence from anesthesia following intubation where coughing is to be avoided; for example, following tonsillectomy or in neurosurgical cases
4. Contraindications:
   - Patients at risk of aspiration (e.g. severe reflux disease, hiatus hernia)
   - Patients difficult to ventilate due to body habitus or chest wall deformity
   - Its use is surgery dependent; for example, the use of an LMA is ill advised in shared airway and laparoscopic surgery (especially in an OSCE)
   - Prolonged surgery, where effective control and manipulation of ventilation may be required
5. The second-generation supraglottic airway devices (SADs) are based on variations of the original LMA. They function in a similar manner but have been designed to include extra features such as integral bite blocks, gastric aspiration ports, introducers and cuff variations (or lack of cuff). Such examples include:
   - ProSeal LMA
   - i-Gel
   - LMA Supreme
   - Laryngeal tube suction mark II

Discussion

- Oropharyngeal and nasopharyngeal airways often are not sufficient to hold open the airway; jaw thrust or chin lift is also needed
- Clearly, an LMA does not protect against airway soiling, so cannot replace a cuffed ETT. Be careful when answering this sort of question that you make this clear
- The original LMA was designed to be reused up to 40 times (washed and sterilized between uses)
- Most SADs now are single use and, while most are variations on a theme of the original, there are a growing number of devices with gastric drainage ports. These are designed to help reduce the risk of aspiration but must be treated with extreme caution – it would not be our recommendation to utilize these in a patient at risk of aspiration

- The cuff pressure on LMAs has been associated with problems other than poor ventilation. There are case reports of patients developing laryngeal nerve palsies attributed to the use of LMAs with the cuff inflated for prolonged periods, transmitting pressure to the nerves through the pharyngeal wall
- Tongue edema has been reported after prolonged use of an LMA or of an oversized LMA

7 Vaporizers

There is almost nothing in anesthesia that cannot be linked to a question about inhaled agents and vaporizers. It is core knowledge and can be examined to demonstrate your understanding of physical principles, pharmacology and clinical anesthesia.

Questions

1. Define the term "vapor."
2. What is the saturated vapor pressure (SVP)?
3. What classes of vaporizers are there?
4. What does "Tec" stand for in the Tec 7 vaporizer?
5. How is this achieved?
6. Which volatile anesthetic agents can be used in a sevoflurane vaporizer?
7. Why does the desflurane vaporizer require electricity to function?
8. What is the pumping effect?
9. What is the Datex–Ohmeda Aladin cassette vaporizer?

Answers

1. A vapor is a gas below its critical temperature, which means that the vapor can be condensed to a liquid by increasing its pressure without reducing the temperature. The critical temperature of a substance is the temperature at and above which vapor of the substance cannot be liquefied, no matter how much pressure is applied.

2. The SVP is the pressure a vapor exerts when the liquid and gas phases are in equilibrium within a closed system at a given temperature. It is temperature dependent up until its boiling point, at which point the SVP is equal to ambient pressure.

3. Broadly, they can be subdivided into *variable bypass vaporizers*, which split the gas flow so that a variable portion of the gas passes through the vaporizer to become saturated with vapor. These can be further subdivided into plenum and draw-over vaporizers. The other type are *measured flow vaporizers*, which produce a saturated vapor that is injected into the fresh gas flow.

4. "Tec" stands for temperature compensated.

5. Temperature compensation can be achieved using a bimetallic strip that adjusts the splitting ratio of the gas flow based on the ambient temperature. At higher temperatures, when more liquid will be vaporized, the amount of gas flow through the vaporization chamber is reduced and vice versa.

6. Only sevoflurane can be used in a sevoflurane vaporizer. The vaporizer is calibrated based on the SVP of the volatile agent for which it is to be used. If a different volatile agent is used, the percentage of gas dialed up and the percentage delivered may be completely different.

7. The desflurane vaporizer is a measured flow device. Desflurane vaporizers are electrically heated to 39 °C, which increases the vapor pressure in the sump to 1300 mmHg, preventing the possibility of boiling in warm operating rooms.

8. When positive pressure ventilation is used, the gas in the circuit is pressurized; this produces back pressure, which is transferred to the vaporizer. Gas in the vaporizer outlet could be forced back into the vaporizing chamber and fully saturated gas from the chamber pushed into the inlet and thence into the bypass channel of the fresh gas flow. This results in delivery of a higher vapor concentration than dialed. Compensating devices in the vaporizer can prevent this occurring.

9. This is a plenum vaporizer with a completely electronic control. The vaporizer settings are controlled from the anesthetic machine control panel, a required concentration can be entered and the vaporizer will adjust the amount delivered to match the input value.

Discussion

- Critical temperature is the temperature above which no increase in pressure can convert the gas back to a liquid
- Draw-over vaporizers are the original type of vaporizer and are located inside the circuit. The patient's respiratory effort draws gas through the vaporizer. Therefore, they have to have an internal resistance low enough to allow the peak inspiratory flow of a breathing patient (usually not more than 60 L/min)
- Plenum vaporizers have a higher internal resistance – too high for draw-over and thus are located outside the circuit.

- A common measured flow vaporizer is the desflurane vaporizer (Tec 6 and variants). This heats the desflurane to 39 °C, well above its boiling point of 23 °C, and this is delivered into the fresh gas flow
- The bimetallic strip works by bonding together two different metals with different coefficients of expansion. Thus the strip bends with changes in temperature. The end can be connected to a valve or inlet such that under cold conditions the strip bends to open the inlet, allowing more gas to flow through the chamber, and vice versa
- The classic question is about similarity in the SVP: halothane and isoflurane have similar SVPs (243 mmHg and 238 mmHg, respectively); therefore, they could theoretically be used in the same vaporizer. **But** this is not advised!
- Halothane requires the addition of the preservative thymol. The vaporizer has to be cleansed of residual thymol on a regular basis to prevent build-up
- An alternative desflurane vaporizer could be one that keeps the desflurane below boiling point and vaporizes it in the same manner as the other volatiles. However, this would not be a fail-safe design; if the cooling device broke, and this failure went undetected, the desflurane could boil in the vaporizer, delivering an enormous – potentially fatal – inspired concentration of desflurane
- The Aladin cassette consists of two parts: the agent-specific vaporizing chamber (the cassette) and the central processing unit (CPU), which is an integral part of the anesthetic machine. It behaves as both a variable bypass and measured flow vaporizer

8 Scavenging

Scavenging is a dry topic but it is a crucial safety system. Never forget to check its working, and do not work without it.

Questions

1. What does a scavenging system do?
2. What are the key components of a scavenging system?
3. Why is the receiving system open to air?
4. How did older passive scavenging systems work?
5. What are the allowed exposure limits for nitrous oxide in the USA?
6. What are the potential risks of chronic nitrous oxide and volatile anesthetic agent exposure?
7. Name some situations where exposure is more likely.

Answers

1. Scavenging systems extract waste anesthetic gases and deliver them outside into the atmosphere to prevent exposure to operating room personnel.
2. A collection system, a transfer system, a receiving system and a disposal system.
3. If the receiving unit were not open to air, the patient would be connected directly to the tubing to the exhaust pump and could suffer respiratory injury.
4. Passive scavenging systems consisted of a sealed canister filled with activated charcoal connected to the collection system. As it absorbs waste gases it gets heavier; thus, when it reaches a certain weight, it has to be replaced. Activated charcoal cannot absorb nitrous oxide. This system is no longer recommended as a permanent scavenging solution.
5. The safe limit for nitrous oxide in the operating environment is 25 parts per million (ppm). Conversion for nitrous oxide, 1 ppm = 1.80 mg/m^3.
6. The evidence is inconclusive although there is a suggestion of an increased risk of spontaneous abortion and congenital abnormalities.
7. Higher levels of exposure to anesthetic gases may be found in:
   - Pediatric operating rooms as a result of gas inductions and non-cuffed endotracheal tubes
   - Post-anesthesia care units (PACUs) where patients exhale anesthetic gases
   - Dental units – where nitrous oxide anesthesia may be obtained via masks

Discussion

- Absorption systems have been used in the past but these are no longer recommended for regular use
- Components of a scavenging system are:
  . Collecting system: for instance, the adjustable pressure limiting (APL) valve gas outlet
  . Transfer system: the hosing connected to the APL gas outlet that transfers the gas to a receiving unit (30-mm tubing to prevent accidental connection to the breathing circuit)
  . Receiving unit: this acts as a reservoir to collect exhaled gases
  . Disposal system: usually an exhaust pump located outside the hospital. This creates a negative pressure, thus generating a constant gas flow through tubing connected from the receiving unit to the pump. It is a high-flow, low-pressure system

- Nitrous oxide and all the halogenated agents are also greenhouse gases
- The receiving unit has a flow indicator, normally a floating cap, to indicate that there is gas flow
- Obstetric units and PACU areas can be made safer simply by having efficient air-conditioning or air-handling systems

9 Medical Gases

The supply of medical gases is another enormous topic. Unfortunately you will have to commit to memory the different sizes and colors of cylinders, pressures and forms in which gases are stored. It may be useful to think back to the physics of pressure before entering the station.

Questions

1. What are oxygen cylinders made of?
2. What pressure exists in a half-full size E oxygen cylinder? What volume of oxygen remains?
3. What pressure exists in a half-full size E cylinder of nitrous oxide? What volume of nitrous oxide remains?
4. What is the filling ratio and why is it important?
5. What is contained in a Heliox cylinder?
6. What is the pin–index safety system?
7. What are the key features of a cryogenic bulk oxygen storage system?
8. What safety features are there to prevent the incorrect gas being piped to the anesthetic machine?

Answers

1. Cylinders can be made of a range of different materials. Traditionally, they were made of carbon steel; now they are often made of molybdenum steel.
2. Oxygen cylinders are filled with compressed gas. As the cylinder empties, the pressure reading will drop in proportion to the remaining volume of gas. A full size E cylinder contains 660 L of gas at 2,200 pounds per square inch (psi). A half-full cylinder would contain 330 L at 1,100 psi.
3. This is a slightly trickier question to answer. Nitrous oxide is in liquid form in the cylinder with a gas layer above; as the cylinder is opened, the liquid undergoes vaporization to maintain the gas layer. If the cylinder is being emptied slowly, the pressure reading will not change from 750 psi (full) until it is nearly empty. If it is being emptied quickly, there will not be enough heat in the volume of liquid nitrous oxide to supply an adequate latent heat of vaporization to keep the gas layer at 750 psi. In this case, the pressure reading will be unpredictable. In either case, a half-full size E cylinder of nitrous oxide contains 800 L. For further reading, compare the critical temperature and critical pressure for oxygen and nitrous oxide.
4. The filling ratio is defined as the weight of substance in the cylinder to the weight of water the cylinder could contain. This is an issue for nitrous oxide (and carbon dioxide) because it is stored as a liquid in cylinders. There has to be a gas space at the top of the cylinder. If there is a very small gas space then slight increases in ambient temperature could cause a dramatic increase in the gas pressure in the gas space, potentially causing the cylinder to explode. The filling ratio for nitrous oxide in temperate climates is 0.75. The critical temperature for nitrous oxide is 36.5 °C. At 20 °C, the saturated vapor pressure of nitrous oxide is 750 psig.
5. Heliox is a mixture of helium 70% and oxygen 30%. It affects gas flow in two ways: the Reynold's number is lower (because density is lower) and thus flow is more likely to be laminar; and if flow is turbulent, resistance to flow will be lower, because Heliox is less dense (~ 0.5 g/L versus 1.2 5 g/L).
6. The pin–index safety system is a safety feature designed to prevent connection of a cylinder containing one substance to a delivery system labelled as a different substance. For example, attaching a nitrous oxide cylinder to the oxygen delivery system would produce 100% nitrous oxide, while you may believe you are attempting to give 100% oxygen. In the past, people have died because of errors of this nature. The system works by having a series of holes drilled into the valve on top of the cylinder in particular positions for each gas – these correspond to pins on the equipment, which prevent connection unless the pins fit into the holes. This is illustrated as follows:

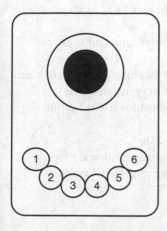

Nitrous oxide	3	5
Oxygen	2	5
Air	1	5
Carbon dioxide	1	6

7. The cryogenic bulk oxygen storage in a hospital setting has the following key features:
- An internal temperature of –160 to –180 °C at a pressure of 10 atmospheres
- An outer shell made of carbon steel and an inner shell made of stainless steel
- A blow-off valve to release excess pressure
- A pressure-raising vaporizer that heats the liquid oxygen to produce gaseous oxygen in times of increased usage. For further reading, review the critical temperature and critical pressure for oxygen
- A pivot or method of weighing the cryogenic storage tank to ascertain how full it is
- Connections to a pipeline distribution system with pressure control panels and safety shut-off valves

8. The Diameter Index Safety System (DISS) for pipeline gases is used, which prevents piped gases from the wall being accidentally connected to the wrong inlet on the machine.

Discussion

- Traditional low-carbon steel is heavy; the newer molybdenum steel cylinders are lighter and stronger. There are even newer composite cylinders, often called "hoop wrap." As the name implies, they are made of a composite of different high-strength and light-weight materials such as steel or aluminium wrapped in Kevlar or carbon fibre
- For oxygen cylinders, the volume they contain is doubled for each alphabetical increase in cylinder size; for example, a C contains 170 L, D 340 L, E 660 L
- Heliox is a mixture of 70% helium and 30% oxygen. It is used for upper airway obstruction to increase laminar flow in the upper airways. Some anesthetic machines come with rotameters designed for Heliox so that gas induction with volatile Heliox is

possible. It should not be used in a patient who requires a higher FiO_2, as its use may produce hypoxemia

- The gas phase of oxygen above the liquid in a cryogenic storage tank and is down-regulated to a pipeline pressure of 50 psi to the hospital
- The vacuum insulator is designed to keep the oxygen liquid. No insulator is perfect and heat will creep in; however, during normal use, draw-off of oxygen causes the temperature of the liquid oxygen to drop as it uses its own heat for latent heat of vaporization to maintain the gas layer
- Oxygen boils at –183 °C and has a critical temperature of –118 °C
- Most hospitals have a supply of oxygen that can last 14 days under normal usage conditions. The vacuum insulated evaporator (VIE) system can deliver oxygen at 3,000 L/min

10 Filters

Heat and moisture exchange (HME) filters have been used in anesthetics for a number of years and confer many benefits to a patient under anesthesia. This is a simple topic that has been asked in examinations numerous times.

Questions

1. What levels of temperature and humidity are normal in the oropharynx?
2. What problems can be caused by dry inspired gases?
3. Explain how an HME device works.
4. What sorts of filters are commonly added to HME devices?
5. What problems can be caused by HME devices?

Answers

1. Temperatures in the oropharynx range between 30 °C and 37 °C, depending on where it is measured. Absolute humidity levels range from 28 to 32 g/m^3. There tends to be a so-called "isothermic boundary" just below the carina; this is the spot at which the inspired gas achieves a temperature of 37 °C and a 100 percent saturation, giving an absolute humidity of 47 g/m^3.

2. Anesthetic gases are waterless (to prevent corrosion), thus leading to mucosal dehydration and impaired ciliary function, impaired surfactant function, inspissation, atelectasis, and an increase in the A–a gradient. There is an increase in the viscosity of the mucus, which slows and then arrests mucociliary transport. Once this happens, cilia stop beating and cell damage occurs. This can cause decreased compliance and loss of functional residual capacitance, atelectasis and shunt. (However, a small [< 400 ppm] amount of water is maintained in sevoflurane to limit degradation by Lewis acids and production of hydrogen fluoride.)

3. An HME device conserves the patient's exhaled heat and moisture. It contains a piece of material coated with a hygroscopic salt such as calcium chloride. Expired gas cools as it passes over this layer, causing water to condense. The water is absorbed by the hygroscopic salt and heat is retained in the material. As the dry inspiratory gas passes over the layer, the heat on the filter warms the gas, and the water molecules bound to the salt are released, increasing the humidity. Maximum efficiency is about 80 percent.

4. The composition of HME filters is very varied; one such example includes fibers that are formed into a nonwoven sheet. This sheet is pleated to give a large surface area and then fitted into a reasonably sized device. Alternatively, filters can be electrostatically charged and generally these do not need to be pleated.

5. HME filters do have disadvantages, which include:
   - Increased resistance to gas flow and hence increased work of breathing
   - Increase in dead space
   - Blockage with secretions and impaired ventilation
   - Unsuitable for long-term prolonged ventilation

Discussion

- Electrostatic filters can be tribocharged or fibrillated coronal-charged filters

  - *Tribocharged filter*: two dissimilar fibers are rubbed together; one becomes negatively charged and one positively charged (cf. your shoe and a carpet on a dry day, leading to static build-up)
  - *Fibrillated coronal-charged filter*: charge is applied to a sheet of material using a point electrode; an opposite charge can be induced on the rear of the sheet. The sheet is stretched and split into fibers (fibrillated) and then made into a nonwoven wad

- Electrostatic filters have less material and so present less of a resistance to breathing

11 Ventilators

Despite familiarity with ventilators and modes of ventilation, it is still easy to become entangled in the jungle of overlapping terminology that surrounds this topic. Mechanical ventilators have become increasingly sophisticated and have outgrown the old classification systems. More important is clinical knowledge of the advantages and disadvantages of the various modes and settings of modern ventilators in both the operating room and intensive care environments. Remember that noninvasive ventilation may also arise in the examination.

Questions

1. Explain how ventilators may be classified in terms of cycling.
2. Explain the difference between pressure and volume control.
3. Draw the pressure–time and flow–time curves produced during pressure-controlled ventilation.
4. Explain the differences between CMV, SIMV and pressure support.
5. What is PEEP?
6. Outline the ventilation strategy for a patient with adult respiratory distress syndrome (ARDS).

Answers

1. This is an old classification system based on how the ventilator cycles from inspiratory to expiratory phases. Ventilators could be time, flow or volume cycled.
2. Volume control: a predetermined volume is programmed into the ventilator and ventilation stops once this volume is achieved. Pressure mode: a predetermined pressure is set; the volume delivered can be highly variable but the ventilator takes no account of this.
3.

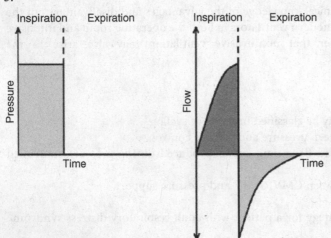

4. CMV is continuous mandatory ventilation: a pressure or volume target is set – also a respiratory rate (frequency) and possibly inspiratory–expiratory times. The ventilator delivers these parameters with no regard for patient effort. SIMV is synchronized intermittent mandatory ventilation: similar parameters are set but, if the patient takes a breath, the ventilated breath can be triggered earlier to support the patient's own effort. Pressure support is designed to allow patients to continue to breathe spontaneously but each breath is detected by the ventilator, which then triggers, giving a predetermined pressure boost to the patient's own respiratory effort.
5. PEEP is positive end expiratory pressure. It is a continuous expiratory pressure designed to prevent collapse of alveoli. This is crucial in diseased lung states and PEEP requirements can range from 0 cmH₂O to 20 cmH₂O.
   Incomplete expiration prior to the initiation of the next breath causes progressive air trapping (hyperinflation). This accumulation of air increases alveolar pressure at the end of expiration, which is referred to as auto-PEEP or intrinsic PEEP.
6. The recommended ventilatory parameters are based on calculating predicted ideal body weight to achieve a tidal volume of around 6 mL/kg with plateau pressures below 35 cmH₂O. This has been shown to improve mortality and reduce the incidence of volutrauma when compared with tidal volumes of 12 mL/kg (ARDSnet study). PEEP values may need to be as high as 24 cmH₂O in order to maintain adequate oxygenation. Hypercapnia should be permitted, within reason. Some intensivists may favor the use of airway pressure release ventilation (APRV), but do not get bogged down with this unless you know exactly how it works.

Discussion

- These old classification systems really are totally irrelevant now but may be around for years to come in examinations
- Different modes of ventilation should be comfortable territory for you with the various advantages and disadvantages tripping off your tongue
- Pressure support mode normally has an automatic apnea override (backup rate) whereby if the patient fails to trigger any breaths, the ventilator will continue ventilation
- ARDS is characterized by:
  - Acute onset respiratory failure
  - Bilateral infiltrates on chest radiograph
  - Non-cardiogenic pulmonary edema
  - $PO_2:FiO_2 < 300$ mmHg

Ventilation is often difficult and aggressive ventilation parameters designed to normalize physiology can result in barotrauma, volutrauma and atelectasis.

ARDSnet is a research group that conducts clinical trials on ARDS and provides evidence-based recommendations on management.

Further Reading List

Al-Shaikh B, Stacey S. *Essentials of Anaesthetic Equipment*, 2nd edn. Churchill Livingstone, 2002.

Banks A, Hardman J. Nitrous oxide. *Contin Educ Anaesth Crit Care Pain*, 2005; 5: 145–148.

Barash P, Cullen BF, Stoelting RK et al., editors, *Clinical Anesthesia*, 6th edn. Lippincott Williams & Wilkins, 2009.

Boumphrey S. Understanding vaporizers. *Contin Educ Anaesth Crit Care Pain*, 2011; 11: 199–203.

Cook T, Howes B. Supraglottic airway devices: recent advances. *Contin Educ Anaesth Crit Care Pain*, 2011; 11: 56–61.

Davey JA, Diba A. *Ward's Anaesthetic Equipment*, 5th edn. Elsevier Saunders, 2005.

Hutton P, Cooper GM, James FM, Butterworth JF. *Fundamental Principles and Practice of Anaesthesia*. Martin Dunitz, 2002.

Miller RD, Eriksson LA, Fleischer LA, Wiener-Kronish JP, Young WL. *Miller's Anesthesia*. 7th edn. Churchill Livingstone Elsevier, 2010.

Wilkes AR. Heat and moisture exchangers and breathing system filters: their use in anaesthesia and intensive care. Part 1 – History, principles and efficiency. *Anaesthesia*, 2011; 66: 31–39.

Wilkes AR. Heat and moisture exchangers and breathing system filters: their use in anaesthesia and intensive care. Part 2 – Practical use, including problems, and their use with paediatric patients. *Anaesthesia*, 2011; 66: 40–51.

1 Electricity

The philosopher Wittgenstein once wrote "whereof one cannot speak, thereof remain silent"; however, Wittgenstein never had to take an OSCE. Here you need to say **something** sensible even if you do not really know. Hazard symbols are easy to examine but tedious to learn. It is highly unlikely you will be presented with an entire station on hazards but they may well be scattered among the relevant clinical stations.

Questions

1. What are the potentially harmful effects of electric current passing through the body?
2. What is the frequency of alternating current (AC) current?
3. What magnitude of alternating current is required to produce:
   (a) Pain
   (b) Muscle contraction
   (c) Ventricular fibrillation (VF)
4. What is "microshock"?
5. How do we prevent shocks in the operating room setting?
6. What do these safety symbols represent?

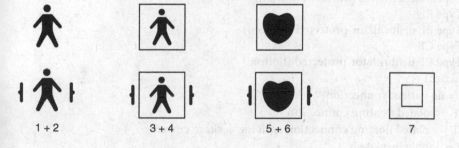

1 + 2   3 + 4   5 + 6   7

Answers

1. Electrocution, ventricular tachycardia, death, burns (resistors heat up when current flows across them), electrochemical effects (excitable tissues such as muscle or nerves can be stimulated) and ignition of flammable materials (e.g. alcoholic skin preparation).

2. North America uses a frequency of 60 Hz, most commonly combined with 110–120 volts. If two-phase AC is used, the voltage is 220–240 volts.

3. The magnitudes of current required are as follows:

Pain	5 mA
Muscle contraction	15–20 mA
Ventricular fibrillation	100 mA

4. Microshock occurs when medical devices that have electrodes in or around the heart (e.g. a Swan–Ganz catheter) are utilized and a current can potentially pass directly to the heart. Here a current as low as 100 µA can cause VF.

5. Most shocks occur as a result of unwanted current returning to ground through the patient; thus, safety strategies are devised to minimize this occurrence. The options are:
   (a) An isolating transformer either for the whole of the operating room or integrated into each electrical device, and
   (b) A ground fault circuit interrupter (GFCI) or an appliance leakage current interrupter (ALCI)

6. These pictures denote various classes and types of electrical equipment.
   1 – Type B
   2 – Type B defibrillator protected (bottom)
   3 – Type BF
   4 – Type BF defibrillator protected (bottom)
   5 – Type CF
   6 – Type CF defibrillator protected (bottom)
   7 – Class II

   Type B = no patient connection
   Type BF = isolated floating connection
   Type CF = isolated floating connection with low-leakage current
   Class II = doubly insulated

Discussion

- Direct current (DC) and AC can cause similar harmful effects to the human body although AC is more dangerous for similar current flows. DC shock tends to cause single muscle spasm with the victim being "blown away" from the shock whereas AC produces tetany (at frequencies of 40–110 Hz), and as the flexor muscles are usually stronger than the extensors, this means the victim may be unable to let go of the source of shock
- Ironically, the frequency best adapted for efficient power transfer in national grids is also in the range most fatal to humans. The following table summarizes the effects of AC at different magnitudes

- The isolating transformer has an output that is free from earth: if any earth leakage occurs it is detected by a relay, which trips the circuit. This type of system is termed "fully floating"

Current (mA)	Effect
1	Tingling
5	Pain
15	Muscle contraction and severe pain
30	Last chance to "let go"
50	Contraction of respiratory muscles leading to asphyxia
70	Cardiac failure, ectopic beats, dysrhythmias
100	Local burns, VF
1,000	Extensive, severe burns

2 Lasers

Laser surgery is becoming increasingly popular so a thorough knowledge of the physics and safety of laser practice is required. This station may also involve a discussion about laser tubes and specific requirements for laser surgery.

Questions

1. What does the acronym LASER mean?
2. What are the benefits of using lasers in clinical practice?
3. What are the potential hazards of laser use in the operating room?
4. How are these hazards mitigated?
5. Name some different types of laser and their specific surgical uses
6. What does Nd–YAG stand for?
7. How would you manage an airway fire in an intubated patient?

Answers

1. Light Amplification by Stimulated Emission of Radiation.
2. The laser allows power to be focused at a very small area as either a cutting device or as a coagulation/ablation device. This enormous amount of energy focused on a small area means that laser surgery offers a near bloodless field.
3. Hazards can be divided into patient hazards and personnel hazards.
   Patient hazards:
   - Accidental vessel or viscus perforation (blood vessels > 5 mm diameter cannot be coagulated by laser)
   - Venous gas embolism (often by the coolant gas used at the laser tip)
   - Laser fires – surgical drapes and anything in contact with flammable skin preparations can be ignited
   - Airway fires – if an endotracheal tube (ETT) is ignited, the consequences are catastrophic, usually resulting in death
   Personnel hazards:
   - Laser plume inhalation (similar to electrocautery smoke inhalation)
   - Accidental eye damage due to reflected laser beams
4. Again, these can be divided into patient and personnel considerations.
   Patient considerations:
   - Laser ETT packed with water-soaked swab
   - Avoid nitrous oxide
   - Low concentrations of inspired oxygen
   Personnel considerations:
   - Adequate safety briefing
   - Laser safety officer for operating rooms
   - Wavelength-specific safety goggles
   - Blinds for the operating room windows
   - Adequate signage that laser surgery is underway in the operating room
   - All instruments and exposed surfaces should have a matte finish to prevent reflection of laser beams
5. The various types of laser you may come across are as follows:
   Ruby laser:
   - Red, 694 nm
   - Used in ophthalmic surgery
   Carbon dioxide laser:
   - Wavelength 10,600 nm, far infrared light
   - Penetrates tissues up to a depth of 2 mm
   - Used for coagulation and cutting in superficial surgery and has roles in neurosurgery, ear, nose and throat (ENT) surgery and dermatology
   Argon laser:
   - Wavelength 450–700 nm, blue-green light
   - Absorbed by hemoglobin but not by aqueous or vitreous humor
   - Used in ophthalmology and dermatology for photocoagulation
   - Replacement for the ruby laser

Nd–YAG laser
- Wavelength 1,064 nm, near infrared
- Penetrates 80–120 mm into tissues, not absorbed by water
- Used for photocoagulation and debulking of tumors and can also be used endoscopically

6. Neodymium–yttrium aluminum garnet (Nd–YAG)
   This is a solid rod laser that uses a photoflash to excite the atoms within the rod to produce a laser beam.

7. Management must be rapid, well-rehearsed and is outlined below. Laser fires are often catastrophic and carry an extremely high mortality rate:

- **Stop** the procedure, turn off all gases and call for help
- **Extinguish** the fire using water or saline, soaked swabs and remove any debris from the airway under direct vision
- **Remove** the ETT and inspect it for damage, burns and patency (some material may still be stuck within the trachea)
- Hand ventilate with 21% oxygen initially then 100% oxygen once the fire is fully extinguished
- Direct laryngoscopy, bronchoscopy or rigid bronchoscopy should be performed and the airway secured with re-intubation of the trachea
- Further cold saline lavage of the airway
- If severe, as is often the case, consider:
  - Arterial line and blood gases
  - Chest X-ray
  - Intensive care involvement
  - ENT opinion with possible early tracheostomy
  - Repeat bronchoscopy
  - Possible extracorporeal membrane oxygenation (ECMO)

Discussion

- Laser light is a coherent, collimated beam of pure monochromatic light. The wavelength is determined by the lasing medium used. In turn, different wavelengths of laser light have various clinical uses because of their different tissue absorbance
- Laser light is produced by an energy pump (e.g. a high-voltage or a xenon flash lamp), which provides the energy to stimulate population inversion of orbital electrons in the material of the lasing medium and a pair of axial mirrors at each end of the lasing tube that allow maximum amplification by stimulated emission of collimated photons. One of the mirrors is not completely reflective, thus allowing the beam to escape; it is then focused and channeled to the patient
- The laser does not increase the power of photons reaching the tissue; it simply allows a colossal number of them to be directed into one very small area
- Some lasers are pulsed so as to minimize the heating effect of tissue around the target area. A technique called "Q-switching" allows laser light to be stored and then released in bursts of higher energy. This is used in retinal laser surgery to prevent thermal damage to the eye

3 Positioning

This is unlikely to represent a genuine OSCE station but is a "catch-all" designed to focus awareness on common hazards such as patient positioning and human factors in critical situations.

Questions

1. What are the three most common nerves injured as a result of patient positioning during surgery?
2. What risk factors are associated with perioperative peripheral nerve injury?
3. What are the signs and symptoms of ulnar nerve damage?
4. What areas may be injured during lithotomy positioning on the operating table?
5. What are the hazards of the prone position?
6. How can the anesthesiologist reduce the incidence of perioperative peripheral nerve injury?
7. What is bone-cement implantation syndrome?
8. In relation to clinical errors, what are human factors?

Answers

1. The three most common nerve injuries involve the:

   - Ulnar nerve (30%)
   - Brachial plexus (20%)
   - Lumbar plexus (15%)

2. Risk factors can either be surgical, anesthetic or patient related.

   Surgical:
   - Use of tourniquets, tight casts or dressing
   - Use of retractors, cutting and compression of nerves
   - Orthopedic, cardiac, maxillo-facial and neurosurgery
   - Surgery specific positioning, i.e. lateral, arms out, reverse Trendelenberg, lithotomy

   Anesthetic:
   - Poor positioning
   - Inadequate padding and protection of extremities
   - Regional anesthesia
   - Hypothermia
   - Hypotension

   Patient:
   - Male
   - Obese or underweight
   - Advanced age
   - Pre-existing neuropathy
   - Diabetes, smoking, peripheral vascular disease

3. A patient with ulnar nerve damage may complain of altered sensation over the medial one and a half digits of the hand. This includes paresthesia, anesthesia, hyperesthesia and pain. Weakness of the intrinsic muscles of the hand may ensue and in severe ulnar nerve damage produce the ulnar "claw hand." Patients may show signs of muscle atrophy, soft-tissue swelling, loss of hair, cutaneous flushing, severe pain and underlying osteoporosis, all of which suggest progression to complex regional pain syndrome. The distribution of the sensory/motor deficit will ultimately depend on where the ulnar nerve has been damaged. The most common site of injury is at the level of the elbow as the nerve passes through the condylar groove.

4. The common peroneal nerve winds around the head of the fibula and may be impinged by a lithotomy pole. This is less of a hazard with modern lithotomy "boots" rather than slings. Lithotomy flattens the lumbar lordosis and may cause worsening of lumbar spine pain. Prolonged lithotomy, especially if accompanied by periods of hypotension, can cause ischemia of the calf muscles secondary to hypoperfusion and a rebound compartment syndrome in the postoperative phase, due to ischemic inflammation. There may also be damage to the sciatic nerve following long surgical procedures.

5. Prone positioning is not to be undertaken lightly as it has many potential problems:

   - The patient must be intubated and the endotracheal tube well secured in the correct position before placing the patient prone. In the event of inadvertent extubation the patient will have to be turned supine again to be re-intubated
   - Ventilation in the prone position may be more difficult and require higher airway pressures and the application of positive end expiratory pressure (PEEP).

Note: prone positioning is thought to increase functional residual capacity (FRC) and improve V/Q mismatch, hence its use in intensive care for refractory hypoxemia and adult respiratory distress syndrome (ARDS).

- Compression of the abdomen can impede venous return
- Ocular damage: direct trauma to the cornea from pressure. The Anesthesia Closed Claim Project has a Postoperative Visual Loss Registry collecting detailed case reports of visual loss after non-ophthalmic surgery. Ischemic optic neuropathy (ION) is one common diagnosis
- Careful attention must be paid to pressure areas – pressure sores can occur on the face, shoulders, elbows and hips
- Monitoring and intravenous access must be appropriately placed and well secured
- Case reports have shown that cardiopulmonary resuscitation (CPR) can be effectively performed to the prone patient. Compressions should be performed on the medial thoracic cage at 100/min

6. As anesthesiologists, we can take steps to help prevent nerve injuries by:

- Identifying patients at high risk
- Avoiding stretching of limbs and over extension of joints
- Ensuring adequate padding of pressure points and elbows
- Avoiding hypotension and maintaining adequate tissue perfusion
- Careful preoperative assessment of patients with pre-existing neurology
- Ultrasound guidance for regional blocks
- Careful application of tourniquets and appropriate inflation pressures

7. A potentially fatal syndrome of unclear pathophysiology related to cemented hip and knee arthroplasty. This often occurs a few minutes after cementing has taken place and is usually characterized by various degrees of hypoxemia associated with dysrhythmias and hypotension. These may be unresponsive to epinephrine or atropine. Death may occur despite immediate and prolonged resuscitative efforts.

8. "Human factors" is a term designed to recognize that humans are fallible and prone to errors. The goal is to identify factors that may cause reduction in performance and highlight ways these can be addressed. These are often referred to as "non-technical skills."

Discussion

- Patient positioning is something we do on a daily basis. More complex positions are associated with higher rates of nerve, joint and tissue damage, so care must always be taken. Areas such as the brachial plexus are often at risk, especially when the arms are positioned perpendicular to the table
- There are multiple theories about the origin of bone-cement implantation syndrome. There are two broad models: the monomer-mediated model and the embolic model
  The *monomer model* postulates that circulating methylmethacrylate (MMA) from the bone cement reaches levels causing critical vasodilatation.
  The *embolic model* focuses on showers of thrombi, fat, bone, fibrin and cement emboli being the cause of the syndrome. These have been demonstrated to occur during cementation using echocardiography and have been demonstrated on postmortem but the degree of embolization seems to correlate poorly with the observed clinical picture.

4 Blood Transfusion

"Yet who would have thought the old man to have had so much blood in him." I'm sure you will have anesthetized the occasional vascular patient where you and Lady Macbeth see eye-to-eye. Remember that there is a good reason why medicine has a whole specialty devoted to the study of blood and its disorders: no one is expecting you to know everything, but a safe, concise knowledge of blood and blood products and the potential hazards of transfusion are essential.

Questions

1. What determines ABO blood grouping?
2. What is meant by the terms "universal donor" and "universal recipient"?
3. In what media can packed red cells be stored?
4. What is prothrombin complex concentrate (PCC)?
5. What is recombinant factor VII?
6. What are the different modes of life-threatening transfusion reactions?
7. What signs of a severe/life-threatening transfusion reaction might a patient under general anesthesia display?
8. What would be your initial management of a severe transfusion reaction?

Answers

1. This is determined by the antigens found on red blood cells (RBCs) and the antibodies in serum against RBC antigens. Therefore:
   - Group A has A antigen on RBCs and anti-B antibodies
   - Group B has B antigen and anti-A antibodies
   - Group AB has A and B antigens and no antibodies
   - Group O has neither A nor B antigen but anti-A *and* anti-B antibodies
2. Universal donor: group O (Rhesus negative), which contains no A or B antigens; Universal recipient: group AB (Rhesus positive) – no antibodies.
3. Suitable media include:
   - SAGM: saline–adenine–glucose–mannitol
   - A-CPD: adenine–citrate–phosphate–dextrose
4. This is a solution designed to be used instead of fresh frozen plasma (FFP) for the reversal of warfarin. It contains all the vitamin K-dependent clotting factors as well as protein S and C.
5. Recombinant factor VII (NovoSeven®) is designed for the treatment of hemophilia. Here, uncontrolled bleeding may be the result of a deficiency in factor VII binding to exposed tissue factor and thus triggering clot formation. NovoSeven® also controls bleeds in hemophilia A or B with inhibitors.
6. Life-threatening transfusion reactions include:
   - Acute hemolytic transfusion reactions
   - TRALI – transfusion-associated lung injury
   - Anaphylaxis
   - Transfusion-associated circulatory overload (TACO)
   - Overt bacteremia and systemic inflammatory response syndrome (SIRS) as a result of transfusing a unit of blood contaminated with bacteria (especially a problem with platelets, which are kept warm and are therefore at greater risk of providing a suitable culture medium)
7. The signs displayed will vary depending on the type of transfusion reaction.
   - SIRS-type response: tachycardia, tachypnea, hypotension, fever
   - TRALI: ARDS-type picture with problematic ventilation, higher airway pressures, hypoxia and increased oxygen requirements
   - Derangement in clotting may be noticed by the surgeons due to increased blood loss, oozing and difficulty in stemming bleeding points. This may represent a disseminated intravascular coagulation-like syndrome
8. A transfusion reaction is a critical situation so your assessment and management should follow an ABC (airway, breathing, circulation) approach:
   - Stop the transfusion, keep the intravenous line patent and call for help
   - Check the airway is patent
   - Auscultate the chest, check vital signs, 100% FiO$_2$ and hand ventilate if necessary
   - Assess the patient's cardiovascular status looking for tachycardia, hypotension, signs of cardiac failure and flushing
   - Treat all adverse signs accordingly
   - Inform the surgeon
   - Recheck the identity of the patient and the blood unit documentation
   - Inform the blood bank

Life-threatening reactions may require emergency resuscitative efforts. These patients will require ICU if they survive.

Discussion

- Packed red cells contain no platelets and each bag has a hematocrit of around 60%. SAGM can be stored for 35 days and A-CPD for 42 days
- All blood is screened for human immunodeficiency virus (HIV), hepatitis B and C, human T-cell lymphotropic virus (HTLV), West Nile virus and syphilis. The following tests are not required for all transfusions but are often performed by blood centers or for special-needs patients: Trypanosoma cruzi (Chagas disease) and Cytomegalovirus (CMV)
- Many hospitals now use PCC rather than FFP as it has been shown to be more clinically effective and cost-effective
- Although NovoSeven has been used in patients with major hemorrhage, its use has been plagued by unwelcome side effects such as deep vein thrombosis (DVT), pulmonary embolism (PE) and myocardial infarct (MI). A hematologist should guide its use
- The Centers for Disease Control and Prevention (CDC) is one of the federal agencies responsible for assuring the safety of the US blood supply by protecting health through investigations and surveillance. The US Food and Drug Administration (FDA) is responsible for regulating how blood donations are collected and blood is transfused. Research on blood transfusion basic science, epidemiology and clinical practices are carried out by the National Institutes of Health (NIH). Keeping the US blood supply safe is also the responsibility of the blood centers and hospitals that collect and transfuse millions of units of blood each year
- Blood transfusion-associated adverse reactions that are tracked through the National Healthcare Safety Network (NHSN) Hemovigilance Module

Further Reading List

Davey JA, Diba A. *Ward's Anaesthetic Equipment*, 5th edn. Elsevier Saunders, 2005.

Donaldson AJ, Thomson HE, Harper NJ, Kenny NW. Bone cement implantation syndrome. *Br J Anaesth*, 2009; **102**: 12–22.

Hardman JG, Contractor S. Injury during anaesthesia. *Contin Educ Anaesth Crit Care Pain*, 2006; **6**: 67–70.

Maxwell MJ, Wilson MJA. Complications of blood transfusion. *Contin Educ Anaesth Crit Care Pain*, 2006; **6**: 225–229.

Miller RD, Eriksson LA, Fleischer LA, Wiener-Kronish JP, Young WL. *Miller's Anesthesia*, 7th edn. Churchill Livingstone Elsevier, 2010.

1 Chest X-Ray 1

Candidate's Instructions

Please look at this X-ray of a 34-year-old intravenous drug user who has presented with acute shortness of breath and a history of nonproductive cough, fever and rigors.

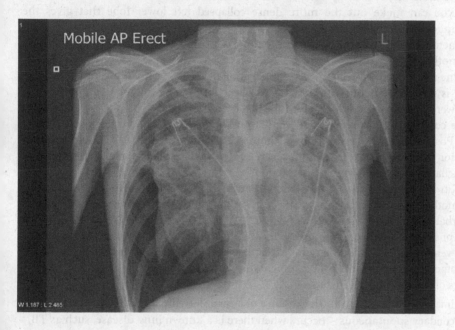

Questions

1. Please interpret this X-ray
2. Is active infection likely?
3. Is there any evidence of left lower lobe collapse?
4. Which abnormality needs immediate management?
5. Can this occur during anesthesia?
6. Is there any evidence of surgical emphysema?
7. What single intervention is required before intubation and ventilation?
8. Is nitrous oxide safe to use in this patient? Why?
9. Why might the patient experience cardiovascular collapse?
10. Give three causes of pneumothorax.

Answers

1. This is a portable anteroposterior (AP) X-ray of the chest. The most obvious abnormalities are a large right-sided pneumothorax with mediastinal and tracheal deviation to the left. There are significant bilateral infiltrates with left upper lobe opacification and left lower lobe collapse.
2. Yes. The history is more important here than the X-ray findings (although they are also suggestive of active infection). This chest X-ray actually demonstrates active tuberculosis (TB) with formation of a cavitating lesion.
3. There is left lower lobe collapse. Although difficult to determine because of mediastinal shift, you can make out the more dense collapsed left lower lobe that gives the appearance of a double heart border.
4. The pneumothorax needs immediate attention as it could quickly progress to a tension pneumothorax.
5. Yes. Pneumothorax is a recognized complication of positive pressure ventilation.
6. There is no subcutaneous emphysema. Surgical emphysema might be more likely if there were rib fractures or if a chest tube had been inserted.
7. Before considering intubating and ventilating this patient, you would insert a chest tube. Positive pressure ventilation without a chest tube in this case could produce a tension pneumothorax, leading to severe cardiovasular collapse, markedly impaired gas exchange and potentially cardiac arrest.
8. No. Nitrous oxide diffuses down its concentration gradient from the blood into the pneumothorax, leading to an increase in volume and pressure within the cavity, exacerbating any tensioning effects.
9. If the pneumothorax were to increase in size, it would cause further mediastinal shift. Thus, venous return would be reduced, cardiac output would fall and the result would be profound hypotension with a compensatory tachycardia.
10. Causes of pneumothorax include:
    - Primary spontaneous – in the absence of any underlying lung disease
    - Secondary spontaneous – occurs when there is a known lung disease, such as TB, chronic obstructive pulmonary disease (COPD), malignancy
    - Trauma – penetrating chest wall injury, rib fractures, blunt trauma
    - Iatrogenic – intermittent positive pressure ventilation, central line insertion, nerve blocks (paravertebral, interscalene, supraclavicular), barotrauma

Discussion

- You may want to comment on the quality of the radiograph, so be systematic in your approach. Things to comment on may include:
  1. Is it an AP or posterioranterior (PA) film?
  2. Is the film adequately penetrated. Are thoracic vertebral bodies visible?
  2. Check the quality of the film. Is it full inspiration, are ten posterior ribs visible?
  3. Is the image rotated? Compare the clavicles and thoracic spine alignment.
  4. Highlight left from right and comment on the gastric bubble if present.

2 Chest X-Ray 2

Candidate's Instructions

This is a chest X-ray of a 72-year-old man who has deteriorated overnight. He is febrile and hemodynamically unstable.

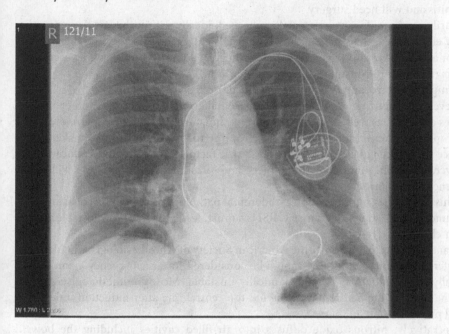

Questions

1. When judging whether a chest radiograph is appropriately exposed what features would you look for?
2. What does this film show?
3. Does this patient's pacemaker need to be checked prior to surgery?
4. Would it be safe to use bipolar electrocautery if this patient needed surgery?
5. What specific equipment would you require before anesthetizing a patient with a pacemaker?
6. Does the presence of the pacemaker alter your antibiotic management?
7. Would a rapid sequence intubation (RSI) be indicated? Why?
8. What monitoring would you want for induction of anesthesia?
9. What issues might there be if using nitrous oxide in this case?
10. Where would you like to send this patient postoperatively?

Answers

1. This film is adequately exposed as you can see the first seven thoracic vertebrae and the hilar vessels clearly.

2. This is an erect anteroposterior (AP) film showing free air under the right hemidiaphragm, suggesting perforation of the gastrointestinal (GI) tract and pneumoperitoneum. There is a pacemaker *in situ* with a fluid-filled bowel loop under the left hemidiaphragm. This man has a perforated viscus and, given the history, he is likely to have peritonitis and will need surgery.

3. Ordinarily you would want a pacemaker checked, ideally within the last three months for any elective case. This patient, however, needs emergency surgery and there is not time for a pacemaker check. Have a magnet available. Some hospitals have a pacemaker technician willing to consult in the operating room.

4. Yes. Unipolar electrocautery should be avoided. Bipolar is acceptable.

5. Whenever anesthetizing a patient with a pacemaker, you should have other pacing facilities available, as well as access to isoproterenol, atropine and glycopyrrolate.

6. No. Prophylactic antibiotics are no longer routine for patients with pacemakers (the presence of a pacemaker is not listed as a risk factor for developing endocarditis). However, given the nature of the surgery and presumed peritonitis, he will need intravenous antibiotics.

7. Yes. This patient has significant intra-abdominal pathology, is at high risk of aspiration and is undergoing emergency surgery. RSI is a must, using the most cardiostable agents of your choice.

8. You want full monitoring as per the American Society of Anesthesiologists' guidelines. The arterial line and central line should be considered for an emergency laparotomy, especially if the patient is hemodynamically unstable. Most anesthesiologists would place the arterial line before induction and the central line after induction unless the clinical picture dictated otherwise.

9. Intraoperatively, nitrous oxide diffuses into air-filled cavities including the bowel. If there is pre-existing bowel obstruction then this may lead to perforation and will exacerbate bowel distension, making surgery more difficult. Postoperatively, it can contribute to intestinal edema, abdominal distension and nausea. As such, it is contraindicated in surgery for acute bowel obstruction and emergency abdominal surgery.

10. Considering the background of a 72-year-old man with a pacemaker undergoing emergency surgery, who may need vasoactive support and ongoing invasive monitoring, regular observations and close fluid balance. The early procurement of a surgical intensive care unit bed will help to avoid delays in the operating room at the end of the case.

3 CT Head

Candidate's Instructions

Please look at this scan of a 62-year-old woman who is admitted through the emergency department.

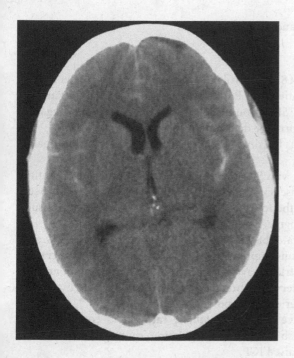

Questions

1. What does this CT scan show?
2. How may this patient present?
3. Give two risk factors for this condition.
4. What percentage of these cases are detectable on a CT scan?
5. Does this patient need a lumbar puncture (LP)?
6. What cardiovascular complications are associated with this condition?
7. Is ketamine a good choice for induction of anesthesia? Why?
8. What are the risks of maintaining anesthesia using a concentration of volatile agent greater than one minimum alveolar concentration (MAC)?
9. Give two respiratory complications associated with this pathology.
10. Give four principles of anesthetic management for this patient.

Answers

1. The scan shows an extensive subarachnoid hemorrhage (SAH) with hydrocephalus.
2. The classical presentation is that of a severe, sudden-onset or "thunderclap" headache associated with signs of meningism such as photophobia, neck stiffness and vomiting. Depending on the severity of the bleed, the patient may demonstrate a fluctuating level of consciousness, seizures and focal neurological deficits.
3. Risk factors associated with SAH include:
   - Presence of cerebral aneurysms
   - Smoking, alcohol consumption and drug abuse
   - Hypertension
   - Family history
4. CT scanning is said to pick up 95% of SAH, with some studies reporting a greater degree of sensitivity. If the CT scan is negative, an LP may be performed looking for xanthochromia of the cerebrospinal fluid (CSF). Around 2–4 percent of people with a negative CT head will have evidence of hemorrhage detected on LP.
5. An LP is not necessary in this case as the diagnosis is clear from the CT! Additionally, there is evidence of hydrocephalus.
6. A significant percentage of patients with SAH have demonstrable ECG abnormalities. They range from arrhythmias to ischemic changes. These disturbances have been attributed to the increase in sympathetic activity that follows the neurological insult. Myocardial infarction (MI) is a recognized complication of SAH.
7. No. Ketamine increases the heart rate, blood pressure (BP), cerebral blood flow and cerebral metabolic rate of oxygen consumption ($CMRO_2$) and thus raises intracranial pressure (ICP). In head injury, one tries to avoid surges in BP and to maintain normal cerebral blood flow in order to preserve cerebral perfusion pressure. Severe hypertension can be just as detrimental as periods of hypotension.
8. Volatile anesthetic agents all reduce cerebral metabolic rate but at concentrations greater than 1 MAC, they can abolish cerebral autoregulation, causing vasodilatation, increased cerebral blood flow and raised ICP.
9. Neurogenic pulmonary edema and aspiration pneumonia.
10. The basic principles of managing a patient with a head injury are to prevent secondary brain injury by optimizing oxygen delivery and reducing demand. This may be achieved by:
    - Maintaining an adequate cerebral perfusion pressure (i.e. > 65 mmHg)
    - Avoiding periods of hypoxia and treating anemia
    - Aggressive treatment of factors that increase cerebral oxygen demand, such as fever, seizures and hyperglycemia
    - Taking steps to help minimize ICP:
      - Ventilate to normocapnia
      - Adequate anesthesia and analgesia to reduce cerebral metabolic rate
      - Avoiding increased venous pressure – head-up tilt, ensure that endotracheal tube ties do not occlude the jugular veins, adequate paralysis to prevent coughing and straining
      - Observing careful fluid balance in an attempt to prevent further cerebral edema
      - Avoiding drugs that increase ICP such as high dose inhalational agents

4 Cervical Spine

Candidate's Instructions

Please look at this X-ray of a 64-year-old woman.

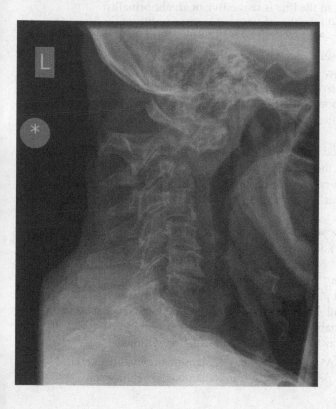

Questions

1. Comment on the adequacy of this film.
2. How is vertebral alignment assessed on a cervical spine X-ray?
3. Describe the major abnormality.
4. Comment on the body of C2.
5. Does this X-ray show significant soft-tissue swelling?
6. Is this likely to be a result of trauma? Why?
7. Why may this pathology be life-threatening?
8. Is the transverse ligament likely to be intact still? Why?
9. Give three conditions associated with this abnormality.
10. What major concerns would you have when anesthetizing this patient?

Answers

1. This is an adequate lateral cervical spine X-ray. An adequate film must include vertebrae C1–C7 with associated anterior structures, the vertebral column in the center of the film and it must extend from the base of the skull down to at least T1.

2. Alignment of the cervical column is assessed using three lines. The anterior vertebral line, the posterior vertebral line and the spinolaminar line. These lines should be confluent. Any deviation from the line is suggestive of an abnormality.

3. This film shows gross instability of the atlantoaxial junction with subluxation of C1 and C2 on C3.

4. The body of C2 is barely visible and has been almost entirely destroyed – in this case through degenerative disease.

5. No. Soft-tissue swelling above the level of C4 that is greater than 50 percent of the diameter of the vertebral body is significant. This is not visible here, although the skin folds of the anterior neck may be mistaken for swelling in the heat of the moment.

6. No. Although trauma is listed as one of the main causes of atlantoaxial instability, it is relatively rare compared to the incidence in those patients with rheumatoid arthritis. In this case, given the history and in the absence of other significant cervical spine abnormalities and lack of soft-tissue swelling, the fracture is pathological and attributable to pre-existing disease.

7. Such instability can be susceptible to even the smallest of traumatic insults. Injury at this level has the potential to damage the phrenic nerve (C3–C5) leading to respiratory compromise and arrest.

8. No. The transverse ligament holds the odontoid process in place posterior to the anterior arch of the atlas. It plays a key role in resisting anteroposterior movement of the atlas with the axis and lower cervical spine. In atlantoaxial subluxation, the transverse ligament is invariably damaged or completely ruptured.

9. Atlantoaxial subluxation may be found in the following conditions:

   • Rheumatoid arthritis (RA) – 70 percent have a demonstrable upper cervical spine abnormality with 20–25 percent having frank atlantoaxial subluxation
   • Down's syndrome
   • Osteogenesis imperfecta
   • Klippel–Feil syndrome

10. This question may not be so open in the OSCE but think about the anesthetic issues surrounding cervical spine fractures.

    • Airway – limited neck movement and the need for cervical spine immobilization make intubation more difficult. Respiratory compromise necessitates immediate intervention. In the emergency setting, rapid sequence intubation (RSI) with inline cervical spine stabilization would be appropriate. For an elective procedure, consider an awake fiber-optic intubation
    • Respiratory system – pre-existing kyphoscoliosis may affect ventilation, as may pulmonary fibrosis and nodules secondary to RA. Think about the need for postoperative ventilation in intensive care
    • Cardiovascular system – if the cause is trauma, be aware of hypotension and bradycardia due to acute spinal shock. Pericardial effusions may be present in RA

- Central nervous system – pre-existing sensory and motor function needs to be assessed

This is by no means an extensive discussion but highlights some of the problems you may face given this scenario.

5 Angiogram

Candidate's Instructions

Please look at the following angiogram. Note that it is taken in the right anterior oblique view.

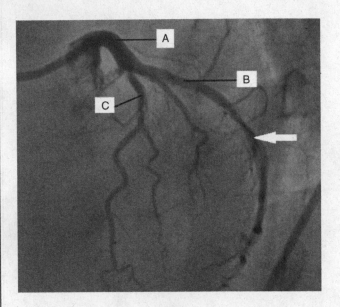

Questions

1. Label structures A, B and C.
2. What ECG changes might you see if there was an acute occlusion at the arrow and in which leads would these changes occur?
3. What areas of the myocardium are supplied by C?
4. What are the sinuses of Valsalva?
5. Which vessels supply the sinoatrial (SA) and atrioventricular (AV) nodes?
6. What is normal coronary blood flow?
7. Give four factors affecting coronary blood flow.
8. Give four risk factors for ischemic heart disease.

Answers

1. A: Left main stem
   B: Left anterior descending (LAD) artery
   C: Circumflex artery

2. The LAD artery supplies much of the myocardium of the left ventricle and, as such, infarcts in this region carry a high mortality. Occlusion would produce characteristic ECG changes of myocardial ischemia and/or infarction, including ST segment elevation or depression, T-wave inversion and later the formation of Q-waves. ECG changes will show ST elevation in V1–4. These changes may be difficult to locate accurately in the presence of a bundle branch block or severe left ventricular hypertrophy with a strain pattern.

3. The circumflex artery supplies the left atrium and the posterolateral wall of the left ventricle. It anastomoses with the interventricular branch of the right coronary artery on the posterior aspect of the heart.

4. The sinuses of Valsalva are also known as the aortic sinuses. They are outpouchings of the ascending aorta that occur just superior to the aortic valve. There are typically three sinuses: right, left and non-coronary. They give rise to the right coronary artery, left main coronary artery and the non-coronary sinus usually contains no vessel origin.

5. The right coronary artery supplies the SA node and also supplies the AV node in 85–90 percent of people.

6. Normal coronary blood flow is approximately 225–250 mL/min or around 5 percent of cardiac output.

7. Factors affecting coronary blood flow are:
   - Vessel diameter and patency (presence of atherosclerosis, factors producing coronary vessel dilatation/constriction)
   - Heart rate (determines duration of diastole, during which time coronary blood flow is greatest)
   - Blood viscosity
   - The pressure gradient between aortic end-diastolic pressure and left ventricular end-diastolic pressure. This is the main determinant of coronary blood flow and, therefore, must be maintained in those with myocardial disease

   Note: some of these factors can be represented by the Hagen–Poiseuille equation

   $$\text{Flow} = \frac{\Delta P \pi r^4}{8 \eta l}$$

8. Risk factors for ischemic heart disease include:
   - Male gender
   - Age
   - Smoking
   - Hypertension
   - Diabetes
   - Obesity
   - Positive family history

1 Cardiovascular Examination

Candidate's Instructions

Examine this patient's cardiovascular system.

Introduction

Develop your own structure and style and become fluent at it. Be confident but not overly so; be calm and friendly towards your patient. Talk to the examiner as you go through the examination, explaining what you are doing, but do not expect any feedback. A suggested structure for a cardiovascular examination is described as follows:

Approach

- Introduce yourself, ask the patient's name and briefly explain what you are going to do
- Not introducing yourself and poor communication will lose you marks

Inspection

- Look at the patient first. Are they lying comfortably in bed?
- Is there obvious peripheral edema or signs of cyanosis?
- If they are young, consider the possibility of congenital heart disease, or even that this may be a normal examination!

Examination

- *Hands* – Are they warm or cool (suggesting a reduced cardiac output)? Is there clubbing or signs of systemic disease such as arthritis or peripheral cyanosis?
- *Radial pulses* – Check the rate and assess for a collapsing (water hammer) pulse. You may consider looking for radioradial or radiofemoral delay. At this point request or take the blood pressure (BP)
- *Eyes* – Is there xanthelasma or corneal arcus? Look for conjunctival pallor suggestive of anemia. You may suggest fundoscopy at this point
- *Face* – Malar flush may represent pulmonary hypertension secondary to mitral valve disease. Look in the mouth for central cyanosis
- *Neck* – Assess the jugular venous pressure (JVP) with the patient at 45 degrees. Normal height is up to 3–4 cm above the manubriosternal angle. Feel the carotid pulse gently, assessing volume and character
- *Chest* – Look for scars from previous surgery and signs of a pacemaker and palpate the apex beat, checking its placement and character
- *Feet* – Inspect for pedal edema and peripheral pulses, if there is time

Auscultation

- Auscultate over the apex, pulmonary, tricuspid and aortic regions, remembering to listen in the left lateral position in expiration (with the bell of the stethoscope) and sitting forwards in expiration for the subtle murmurs of mitral stenosis and aortic regurgitation, respectively
- Listen over the carotid arteries for bruits or murmur radiation
- Listen over the lung bases for evidence of pulmonary edema

Once you have finished your routine, thank the patient. Without pausing, summarize your findings to the examiner, finishing with a differential diagnosis.

State the other tests you would like to perform. Start simply with clinical investigations such as fundoscopy, looking for signs of hypertension (arteriovenous nicking, hemorrhage, aneurysms, etc.); next, the bedside tests you would do (e.g. urinalysis for hematuria, ECG), before listing blood tests and radiological investigations.

If you spend too long moving the patient around, trying to decide if the diastolic murmur is that of mitral stenosis or aortic regurgitation, you will run out of time and score poorly. You need a rapid, practiced routine in which you are explaining what you are looking for to the examiners **as you go along.**

Questions

1. How do you differentiate between the JVP and the carotid pulse?
2. What are the symptoms and signs of aortic stenosis?
3. Name three causes of aortic regurgitation?
4. What are the signs of pulmonary hypertension?

Answers

1. On clinical examination, the JVP is biphasic and is easily occluded by gentle pressure. The JVP also displays a positive hepatojugular reflex (compression of the liver produces a rise in the JVP).

2. Most people with mild to moderate aortic stenosis do not have symptoms, and it is often diagnosed in asymptomatic people by the finding of an easily heard systolic, crescendo–decrescendo murmur, heard loudest at the upper right sternal border (second right intercostal space) and radiating to the carotid arteries bilaterally. Symptoms are usually present in those with severe aortic stenosis, although they can exist in those with mild to moderate severity as well. A common initial presenting symptom is progressive shortness of breath on exertion. Symptoms of severe aortic stenosis include:
   - Syncope
   - Chest pain
   - Heart failure

   Signs of severe aortic stenosis include:
   - Narrow pulse pressure
   - Slow rising pulse
   - Soft second heart sound
   - Left ventricular failure

3. Causes of aortic regurgitation include:
   - Rheumatic heart disease
   - Ankylosing spondylitis
   - Marfan's syndrome
   - Infective endocarditis

4. Signs of pulmonary hypertension include:
   - Loud pulmonary component of the second heart sound
   - Graham Steel murmur of pulmonary regurgitation
   - Right ventricular heave
   - Tricuspid regurgitation, which may reveal itself through giant V-waves in the JVP

2 Respiratory Examination

Candidate's Instructions

Mr. Simpson is scheduled for an elective knee arthroscopy but states he has been short of breath prior to coming into hospital. Please examine his respiratory system and comment on your findings.

Introduction

Respiratory assessment and examination is a core skill for anesthesiologists and, therefore, a well-practiced routine will be expected.

Approach

- Introduce yourself, explain what you are about to do and appropriately expose the patient

Inspection

- Look for inhalers in the room while you count the respiratory rate
- Make sure you do not miss any thoracotomy scars, previous signs of surgery or radiotherapy

Examination

- *Hands* – Look for nicotine stains, clubbing, wasting of the small muscles or peripheral cyanosis. Check for a carbon dioxide retention flap
- *Radial pulses* – Check for rate and character
- *Eyes* – Look for Horner's syndrome (miosis, ptosis and anhydrosis) secondary to an invading malignancy
- *Face* – Check for central cyanosis or the pursed lip breathing of a "pink puffer"
- *Speech* – A hoarse voice may indicate recurrent laryngeal nerve involvement as a result of malignancy
- *Neck* – Assess the jugular venous pressure with the patient at 45 degrees; it is raised and pulsatile in cor pulmonale. Look at the trachea and check for lateral displacement or for signs of tracheal tug
- *Chest* – Note the shape of the chest, looking for evidence of hyperinflation and for use of accessory muscles. Look for scars from previous surgery before beginning a tactile examination. Check chest expansion both from the front and behind. Place your hands on each side of the chest with your thumbs just touching. Ask the patient to take a deep breath in, then all the way out. Reposition your thumbs so that they are just touching in the midline and ask for a maximal breath in. It is on this last breath that an assessment of how your hand moves from the midline is made

Percussion

- Percuss the chest, looking for areas of hyper-resonance and areas of dullness. Compare left with right

Auscultation

- Auscultate the chest, listening for the quality and character of the breath sounds and also for any added sounds. Crackles may be coarse (secretions in larger airways, e.g. pneumonia) or fine (small airway disease, e.g. pulmonary edema, fibrosing alveolitis). Wheeze may be polyphonic (multiple small airway obstruction such as asthma or chronic obstructive pulmonary disease [COPD]) or monophonic (single large airway obstruction)
- Tactile and vocal resonance give the same information; that is, they will help determine whether an area of dullness is due to either pleural effusion (reduced transmission) or consolidation (enhanced transmission)

Repeat the expansion, percussion and auscultation routine on the back, remembering to check for lymphadenopathy from behind while the patient is sitting up.

Other Areas

- *Abdomen* – It is unlikely you will have time to check for pulsatile hepatomegaly although state that you would look for the other signs of pulmonary hypertension or right-sided heart failure, if that is what you suspect
- *Feet* – Check for pedal edema

Once you have completed your examination, state that you would perform bedside spirometry and pulse oximetry and that you would consider arterial blood gas sampling and/or a chest radiograph, depending on your findings.

Questions

1. What causes of COPD do you know?
2. What is one smoking pack-year?
3. What are the indications for long-term oxygen therapy (LTOT)?
4. What are the common pathogens in community-acquired pneumonia?
5. Can you name any prognostic indicators in pneumonia?
6. What is atelectasis and how can it be avoided?

Answers

1. Smoking, occupational exposure (e.g. coal workers' lung) and alpha-1 antitrypsin deficiency.
2. One pack–year is equal to smoking 20 cigarettes (one pack) a day for one year.
3. According to the American Thoracic Society (ATS) guidelines, patients with chronic hypoxemia should usually be prescribed LTOT when the PaO_2 is consistently at or below 55 mmHg or torr). In addition, LTOT can be prescribed when the PaO_2 is 55–59 mmHg, together with the presence of one of either secondary polycythemia or evidence of pulmonary hypertension. Desaturation only during exercise or sleep suggests consideration of oxygen therapy specifically under those conditions.
4. *Streptococcus pneumoniae* is the most common, followed by *Hemophilus influenzae* and *Mycoplasma pneumoniae*.
5. The Infectious Diseases Society of America (IDSA) and ATS guidelines for community-acquired pneumonia in adults recommend use of severity-of-illness scores, such as the CURB-65. A five-point score, one point for each of:

   - Confusion (abbreviated mental test score ≤ 8)
   - Urea > 19 mg/dL
   - Respiratory rate 30 breaths/min or more
   - Systolic BP below 90 mmHg (or diastolic below 60 mmHg)
   - Age of 65 years or older

CURB-65 score 0	Low risk of mortality, not normally requiring hospitalization
CURB-65 score 1–2	Increased risk of death, consider hospital referral and assessment
CURB-65 score ≥ 3	High risk of mortality, requires urgent hospital admission

6. Atelectasis can be defined as the absence of gas from a segment of lung parenchyma. As the partial pressure of dissolved gas in the blood is less than that in the atmosphere, there is a gradual uptake of gas from obstructed, nonventilated alveoli. This results in alveolar collapse. The process can be expedited by use of a high FiO_2 as this is more readily taken up into the blood than nitrogen. Atelectasis can be reduced by splinting open alveoli with positive end expiratory pressure intraoperatively, and postoperatively by promoting optimal breathing through physiotherapy, good analgesia and appropriate humidification of inspired gases.

3 Cranial Nerve Examination

Candidate's Instructions

Mr. Frank is complaining of a headache and visual disturbances following spinal anesthesia. Please examine his cranial nerves.

Introduction

Cranial nerve examination is often considered a daunting task and not something most candidates would enjoy. However, once you have a routine in place it should be a station where you can gain easy points. Practice your routine thoroughly so that you have some motor memory of what is coming next.

Approach

- Introduce yourself, explain what you are about to do and ensure you are sitting comfortably, facing the patient

Examination

I *Olfactory*

- Have you noticed any loss of smell?

II *Optic*

- Have you had any problems with your vision?
- Look at pupil size and position. Assess acuity by asking the patient to read a near vision chart at 1 ft with each eye in turn, using glasses if they wear them normally
- Assess visual fields by telling the patient to cover his right eye and look at your nose. You now place your right index finger out in the periphery of your visual field at a point roughly equidistant between the two of you. Ask the patient if he can see your finger. If he can't, slowly move your hand towards the two of you until he can see your finger. Check superior and inferior quadrants, temporally and nasally, for both eyes
- Check direct and consensual light reflexes and perform the swinging light test looking for a relative afferent pupillary defect

III *Oculomotor*

- Check eye movements in all four directions

IV *Trochlear*

- Supplies superior oblique muscle which, when the eye is fully adducted, moves the eye down

V *Trigeminal*

- Test the ophthalmic, maxillary and mandibular branches with light touch to the face and check motor function by asking the patient to clench his/her teeth while you look for wasting of the masseter muscles

VI *Abducens*

- Supplies lateral rectus, which adducts the eye

VII *Facial*

- Assess motor function by asking the patient to do the following:

  . Raise his eyebrows
  . Tightly shut his eyes
  . Show his teeth
  . Puff out his cheeks

VIII *Vestibulocochlear or auditory*

- Ask about any problems with hearing or balance. A tuning fork may be provided to perform Weber's and Rinne's tests. Rinne's test compares sound conduction through air and bone by placing a ringing fork both next to the auditory canal and against the mastoid process. If the test is positive, the sound is heard loudest when travelling through the air rather than when in contact with the bone, which is the nonpathological state. If the external auditory canal is occluded, the sound will be loudest on bone conduction, implying middle ear disease or wax. In Weber's test, the tuning fork is placed on the middle of the forehead and the sound should be heard equally in both ears. In sensorineural deafness, sound is not detected by the affected ear. In conductive deafness, sound is loudest in the affected ear.

IX *Glossopharyngeal*

- Mainly a sensory nerve providing sensation to the pharynx. It is tested with the vagus nerve

X *Vagus*

- A complex nerve that is vital for normal speech and swallowing. Test by asking the patient to open his/her mouth and say "ahhh" while you look for upwards movement of the uvula. In pathological states it moves to the contralateral side to the lesion

XI *Accessory*

- Innervates the sternomastoid and trapezius muscles. Ask the patient to shrug his/her shoulders against resistance and to turn his/her head against your hand while you observe the sternomastoid on the opposite side to that to which the patient is turning

XII *Hypoglossal*

- Supplies the intrinsic muscles of the tongue. Observe any fasciculations then ask the patient to stick out his/her tongue. Deviation is to the side of the lesion

To complete your examination, state you would want to assess visual acuity and color vision formally, perform audiometry and fundoscopy and examine the peripheral nervous system.

Going through the motions of a cranial nerve examination is not hard, picking up abnormalities will be difficult if you are concentrating on what you have to do next. It is unlikely that you will have to perform fundoscopy or formally assess visual acuity but you should know how to do both these things.

Questions

1. What is the light reflex?
2. What are the signs of a complete third nerve palsy?
3. What are the signs of optic nerve damage?
4. Which nerves supply the superior oblique and lateral rectus muscles?
5. What is Horner's syndrome?

Answers

1. Light falls on the retina, generating electrical impulses that travel first via the optic nerve and then via the optic tract to the lateral geniculate ganglion. From here fibers pass to the Edinger–Westphal nuclei and oculomotor nuclei in the periaqueductal grey matter of the midbrain. The signal continues in the parasympathetic fibers that entwine the oculomotor nerves and stimulate the ciliary ganglion, ciliary nerves and, finally, the pupillary sphincter muscle of each eye.

2. A complete third nerve palsy will lead to unopposed sympathetic innervation (dilated pupil, loss of accommodation reflex) and unopposed superior oblique and lateral rectus muscles (down and out) coupled with ipsilateral ptosis (loss of levator palpebrae superioris).

3. Decreased visual acuity, optic atrophy, a relative afferent pupillary defect (RAPD), decreased color vision and central scotoma (blind spot). A damaged nerve will atrophy, resulting in reduced acuity and a big central blind spot. The swinging flashlight test is looking for an RAPD as less light is detected by an atrophic optic nerve, resulting in pupillary *dilatation* when the light shines on the affected pupil. Remember the loss of color vision for a bonus point.

4. Trochlear and abducens nerves, respectively.

5. Horner's syndrome is interruption of the sympathetic chain and may occur anywhere from its origin in the hypothalamus to the postganglionic fibers. The most common lesions causing Horner's syndrome affect the sympathetic chain along its outflow from C8/T1 to the superior cervical ganglion and include pathologies such as cervical lymphadenopathy, thyroid masses and neck surgery complications. The signs of Horner's syndrome are:

   • Miosis ipsilateral to the site of the lesion
   • Partial ptosis due to loss of sympathetic nerve supply to the levator palpebrae muscle
   • Anhydrosis of the ispsilateral face
   • Enophthalmos due to paralysis of the eyelid tarsus muscles

4 Obstetric Preoperative Assessment

Candidate's Instructions

This woman is due to have an elective cesarean section. Please perform a preoperative assessment.

Introduction

Obstetric assessment should be regarded as being more akin to a history-taking station than a clinical examination station. Using your standard preoperative assessment, you should be able to structure an answer and obtain most of the points. A history, examination and investigations approach should cover most bases, and is needed, even if the plan is for a regional approach, as not every spinal anesthetic is guaranteed success.

Approach

- Introduce yourself, explain what you are going to do and in what order. Be calm and confident; this type of patient is likely to be nervous and may have a number of hidden concerns

History

- A brief obstetric history should be taken, covering previous pregnancies and modes of delivery. Ask specifically about problems during this pregnancy including hyperemesis, back trouble and reflux. Enquire about the date of the last ultrasound scan and what this scan showed (breech, placental position, etc.)
- Take a routine anesthetic history, including previous surgery, general anesthetics and any complications thereof
- Ask about general health and past medical history
- Is it important to exclude any clotting abnormalities and anticoagulant therapy. (**Note**: some women may be taking low molecular weight heparin [LMWH], so be careful.)
- Obtain a full drug history, including any allergies
- Ask about gastro-esophageal reflux and ability to take nonsteroidal anti-inflammatory drugs (NSAIDs)
- Ask about any dentition and problems with mouth opening/neck movements

Examination

Be guided by your findings from the history but ensure you cover the following:

- Assess the patient's airway as there is a higher incidence of difficult intubation in the obstetric population. Note enlarged breasts, which may make laryngoscopy difficult and may therefore suggest the need for a short-handled blade
- Look at the patient's hands and arms to gauge the difficulty of intravenous access
- Examine the patient's back, again to make a judgement as to the difficulty of regional anesthesia. If the patient has a high body mass index (BMI), it is worth saying that you

135

would consider an ultrasound of the back, which may help locate the depth of the epidural or subarachnoid space
- A short but concise cardiovascular examination may be pertinent, and would be mandatory if the patient had a history of cardiovascular disease. At a minimum, feel the pulse, state you would take the blood pressure (BP) if not already checked and look for signs of anemia and peripheral edema

Investigations

- Check the vital signs, looking for BP measurements, heart rate, SpO_2, height and weight
- Routine blood tests of hemoglobin and platelet count are essential, as is a urine analysis. If eclampsia or HELLP syndrome (hemolysis, elevated liver enzymes, low platelet count) is suspected than renal and liver profiles are needed. If she has diabetes mellitus (even if just gestational) a glucose and HbA1c (if not done recently) are required. A type and screen test should also be done
- The results of the antenatal ultrasound scans should be available. Exclude abnormal placentation, especially if the patient had a previous cesarean section
- Urine samples, looking for evidence of proteinuria, are routine
- A mother with significant cardiac morbidity may have had additional tests, such as ECG and echocardiogram

Taking an obstetric history requires a different mindset to other system examinations and should be performed in the same way as any preoperative assessment, using the tools of history, examination and investigations.

Questions

1. What are the advantages of regional anesthesia over general anesthesia for a cesarean section?
2. What are the contraindications for epidural analgesia in labor?
3. What is placenta previa?
4. What is preeclampsia?

Answers

1. Overall, regional anesthesia has been found to have a better safety profile. Specific advantages include:
   - Lower risk of aspiration
   - Lower risk of anaphylaxis
   - More alert neonate promoting early bonding and breastfeeding
   - Improved postoperative analgesia and earlier mobilization
   - Both mother and partner can be present (and awake) at the time of surgery

2. Contraindications include:
   - Maternal refusal
   - Allergy to local anesthetics (rare)
   - Local infection
   - Uncorrected hypovolemia
   - Coagulopathy – exact levels vary and a clinical judgement of the risks and benefits should be made in each case

3. Placenta previa occurs when the placenta implants between the fetus and the cervical os. Diagnosis is usually made by ultrasound, often after a small, painless vaginal bleed. Placenta accreta is when there is abnormal implantation of the placenta into the uterus. In placenta increta the placenta grows into the myometrium and in placenta percreta the placenta grows through the myometrium to the uterine serosa and into the surrounding structures. The anesthetic implication is that the patient is at risk of major hemorrhage, especially if the placenta is anterior and therefore likely to be cut by the obstetrician.

4. Preeclampsia was formerly defined as hypertension and proteinuria (> 0.3 g/L), which develops after 20 weeks' gestation in a previously normotensive and non-proteinuric woman. According to the new American College of Obstetricians and Gynecologists (ACOG) Task Force on Hypertension in Pregnancy guidelines, the diagnosis of pre-eclampsia no longer requires the detection of high levels of protein in the urine (proteinuria), but it may be diagnosed only on the basis of hypertension. Evidence shows that organ problems with the kidneys and liver can occur without proteinuria, and that the amount of protein in the urine does not predict how severely the disease will progress. Prior to this time, most healthcare providers traditionally adhered to a rigid diagnosis of preeclampsia based on blood pressure and proteinuria. Hypertension in pregnancy is diagnosed by either raised absolute values of systolic, mean or diastolic pressures greater than 140, 105 or 90 mmHg, respectively, or an increase in systolic or diastolic BP greater than 30 or 15 mmHg, respectively, measured at two separate times at least four hours apart. Edema is no longer included in the definition but will often be clinically evident. Preeclampsia is a multisystem disease with a variable clinical presentation and remains a major cause of maternal death worldwide. The pathophysiology of preeclampsia is not fully understood but it is thought that failure of placentation occurs early in pregnancy, leading to vascular endothelial cell damage and dysfunction. The endothelial cell damage is thought to lead to release of vasoactive substances that promote generalized vasoconstriction and reduced organ perfusion. Aspirin is frequently prescribed to prevent preeclampsia in high-risk patients. Magnesium sulfate infusions are used to prevent development of seizures and eclampsia.

5 Peripheral Circulation Examination

Candidate's Instructions

This patient is due to have an elective aorto-bifemoral graft inserted but has started complaining of a painful foot. Please examine his peripheral circulation.

Introduction

This is not something you are likely to do during everyday practice and, therefore, it will not be second nature. Keeping it simple and having a structure will be crucial.

Approach

- Again start by introducing yourself, confirming patient identity and explain what you intend to do to the patient

Inspection

- Inspect the patient looking for scars of previous surgery, signs of impaired perfusion such as pallor of the distal limb, paucity of hairs, ulceration or amputation
- Look at the patient's general appearance. Are there any signs of underlying pathologies such as stigmata of diabetes, smoking or hypercholesterolemia?

Examination

- If the history suggests a lower limb problem, consider starting at the abdomen looking for an aneurysm (a possible source of thromboembolism) by palpation and auscultation
- Feel the femoral pulses, comparing one side against the other (do this for all peripheral pulses). Listen for bruits and check for radiofemoral delay (associated with coarctation)
- An irregular pulse may indicate atrial fibrillation as a thromboembolic cause
- Move to the popliteal pulses, felt in the back of the knee with the knee flexed at 90 degrees. Examine the feet, checking both dorsalis pedis and posterior tibial pulses as well as checking capillary refill and comparing temperature bilaterally
- Comparing the hands with the feet may give you an idea as to whether there is a specific blockage to flow or whether the patient has generalized vascular disease with poor circulation to both the upper and lower limbs
- Continue the examination with the hands, remembering to check for radioradial delay (coarctation proximal to left subclavian outflow), and also perform Allen's test
- Check for a collapsing pulse by feeling both the radial and brachial pulses and then rapidly raising the patient's arm vertically upwards. A collapsing (water hammer) pulse will very briefly tap against your fingers because of the rapid run-off

Auscultation

- Auscultate the carotid arteries, listening for bruits. If an extra noise is heard, you will need to listen to the heart to ensure it is not a transmitted murmur
- Routine examination of the heart when asked to assess peripheral pulses is probably not warranted, although it is the first thing you should say you would like to do once you have completed your routine
- For completeness, or if you fail to palpate any of the pulses, ask to use Doppler ultrasound to check that they are present

Questions

1. What abnormalities in arterial pulse character are you aware of?
2. What additional heart sounds do you know and what is their significance?
3. What are the signs of an ischemic limb?
4. What is the ankle–brachial pressure index?

Answers

1. There are several abnormal arterial waveforms described:
   - Slow rising pulse. Characteristic of aortic stenosis and often accompanied by a narrow pulse pressure
   - Collapsing (water hammer) pulse. Classically due to aortic regurgitation but can also be caused by a patent ductus arteriosus or an arteriovenous fistula. There is a brisk upstroke followed by a sudden collapse due to rapid loss of the diastolic pressure. It is usually associated with a wide pulse pressure
   - Pulsus paradoxus. A misnomer, as this refers to an exaggeration of normal physiology. There is a drop in systolic pressure of > 10 mmHg during inspiration and it may occur in severe asthma or pericardial constriction
   - Pulsus alternans. This refers to alternating large and small beats and may be a sign of left ventricular failure ("Then he felt her pulse. There was a strong stroke and a weak one, like a sound and its echo. That was supposed to betoken the end." *Sons and Lovers*, by D. H. Lawrence.)

2. The most common additional heart sounds are the third and fourth sounds although, infrequently, a stenotic valve may give off a "snap" as it opens (e.g. mitral stenosis). A third heart sound is due to rapid left ventricular filling in early diastole and can be found in healthy young adults or in hyperdynamic states. It may also signify left ventricular failure or mitral regurgitation. A fourth sound is due to vigorous atrial contraction filling a noncompliant ventricle. It is a marker of diastolic dysfunction and may be a consequence of left ventricular hypertrophy or aortic stenosis. It is always pathological. It will not be present in atrial fibrillation.

3. The classical signs of an acutely ischemic limb are the six Ps – pale, pulseless, painful, paralyzed, paresthetic (numb) and perishingly cold.

4. Ankle–brachial pressure index is measured using Doppler ultrasound at the brachial and pedal pulses. The systolic pressures are expressed as a ratio, where 0.4–0.9 represents intermittent claudication and critical ischemia has a value of < 0.3.

6 Airway Examination

Candidate's Instructions

Mr. Davies is on your schedule for dental extractions this afternoon. Please assess his airway.

Introduction

This is something that all anesthesiologists should do when seeing patients preoperatively. A poor understanding of the anatomy and routine tests we use to predict a difficult airway will go down very badly with the examiners.

Assessment of the airway can be divided into history, inspection, examination and investigations.

Approach

- Again, introduce yourself, explain who you are and what you intend to do

History

- Ask a few brief questions trying to elicit a history of:
  - Difficult, failed or fiber-optic intubations
  - Acquired disease like rheumatoid arthritis (RA), ankylosing spondylitis, diabetes
  - Iatrogenic problems such as temporomandibular joint surgery, cervical fusion, oropharyngeal surgery or radiotherapy
  - Ask about sleep apnea, change in voice or new swellings around the neck/mouth
  - Ask about problems breathing at night, especially when lying flat
  - Indicate you would look at previous anesthetic records and note any problems!

Inspection

- General inspection of a patient can give you a lot of information. Comment on the patient's appearance and any factors that may indicate airway problems. Look for:
  - Signs of congenital abnormality – Pierre Robin, Down's syndromes, etc.
  - Obesity
  - Overbite, receding chin
  - Obvious neck swellings
  - Short, fat or muscular neck
  - Presence of a beard – difficulty getting a seal for facemask ventilation

Examination

- *Mouth*
  - Assess mouth opening; it should be 3 cm or more (measured between incisors)
  - Check the Mallampati score

. Check for overbite. An inability to protrude the mandible so that the lower incisors cannot pass in front of the upper incisors is associated with difficult intubation
. Assess dental hygiene and ask about loose teeth and dentures
. Take note of macroglossia and microstomia

- *Neck*
  . Assess neck flexion and, more importantly, extension; poor neck extension confers an increased risk of difficult intubation
  . Check the thyromental distance (Patil's test). A distance of > 6.5 cm is classed as normal. Less than 6 cm predicts approximately 75 percent of difficult laryngoscopies
  . You may choose to palpate the trachea and cricothyroid space
  . Check the temporomandibular joint and assess for movement and swelling
  . Look for any signs of previous surgery, thyroid or tracheostomy scars

- *Nose*
  . Some people would check the patency of nostrils and look for a deviated septum if nasal intubation will be required

Investigations

- Investigations are not commonly used as a predictor of difficult intubation. However, in patients who are highly likely to have a difficult airway (i.e. laryngeal cancer, RA, evidence of stridor and hoarse voice), they may become necessary

Questions

1. What is the Mallampati classification?
2. Give three other measurements that may help in predicting a difficult intubation.
3. What investigations might help you in assessing a patient's airway?

Answers

1. The Mallampati classification is used to predict difficult intubation. The score ranges from I to IV and is described as follows:

Class I	Soft palate, uvula, fauces, anterior and posterior pillars visible
Class II	Soft palate, uvula and fauces visible
Class III	Soft palate and tip of uvula visible
Class IV	Hard palate only, no soft palate visible

   Mallampati scores of III or IV are said to carry a higher incidence of difficult intubation.

2. Three other methods of predicting difficult intubation are:

   - Sternomental distance – measured with the neck fully extended and the mouth closed. A distance between the sternal notch and the chin (mentum) of less than 12 cm is associated with difficult intubation
   - Inter-incisor distance – less than 3 cm predicts a difficult intubation
   - Atlanto-occipital distance – seen on imaging the cervical spine; compression of the space may indicate reduced neck movement and confer problematic intubation

     . You may also want to mention thyromental distance, mentohyoid distance (4 cm) and talk about Wilson's scoring system

3. Investigations that one might employ are:

   - Cervical spine X-rays and flexion/extension views can identify unstable cervical pathology such as atlantoaxial instability
   - CT scans or MRI can define the anatomy where severe distortion of the normal anatomy is expected
   - Chest X-rays can sometimes demonstrate a retrosternal goiter that may be compressing the trachea
   - Endoscopic assessment of the airway can also be performed prior to anesthesia to assess suitability for fiber-optic intubation

Further Reading List

British Thoracic Society Working Group on Home Oxygen Services. Clinical component for the home oxygen service in England and Wales. *Thorax*, 2015, **70**: i1–i43.

Crossman A, Neary D. *Neuroanatomy*, 2nd edn. Harcourt Publishers Ltd, 2000.

Hall T. *PACES for the MRCP*. Churchill Livingstone, 2003.

Kumar P, Clark M. *Clinical Medicine*, 5th edn. Elsevier Science, 2011.

Lim WS, Woodhead M, British Thoracic Society. British Thoracic Society adult community acquired pneumonia audit 2009/10. *Thorax*, 2011; **66**: 548–549.

Longmore M, Wilkinson I, Turmezei T, Cheung CK. *Oxford Handbook of Clinical Medicine*, 7th edn. Oxford University Press, 2007.

Mandell LA, Wunderink RG, Anzueto A et al. Infectious Diseases Society of America/American Thoracic Society Consensus Guidelines on the management of community-acquired pneumonia in adults. *Clin Infect Dis*, 2007; **44**: S27–S72. See www.thoracic.org/statements/resources/mtpi/idsaats-cap.pdf.

Preeclampsia Foundation. New guidelines in preeclampsia diagnosis and care include revised definition of preeclampsia. See www.preeclampsia.org/the-news/3-news flash/299-new-guidelines-in-preeclampsia-diagnosis-and-care-include-revised-definition-of-preeclampsia.

Qaseem A, Wilt TJ, Weinberger SE, Diagnosis and management of stable chronic obstructive pulmonary disease: A clinical practice guideline update from the American College of Physicians, American College of Chest Physicians, American Thoracic Society, and European Respiratory Society. *Ann Intern Med*, 2011, **155**: 179–191.

Vaughan RS. Predicting difficult airways. *Contin Educ Anaesth, Crit Care Pain*, 2001; **1**: 44–47.

Whitaker R, Borley N. *Instant Anatomy*, 2nd edn. Blackwell Science, 2000.

Wilson M, Spiegelhalter D, Robertson A, Predicting difficult intubation. *Br J Anaesth*, 1988; **61**: 211–216.

Yentis S, May A, Malhotra S. *Analgesia, Anaesthesia and Pregnancy*, 2nd edn. Cambridge University Press, 2007.

1 Bradyarrhythmia

Candidate's Instructions

Please look at this rhythm strip. The paper speed is 25 mm/s.

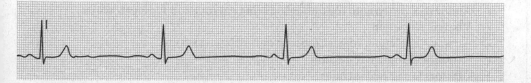

Questions

1. What is this rhythm and what is its first line management?
2. Which surgical interventions commonly cause vagal stimulation?
3. What are the risk factors for asystole?
4. What additional methods are available to treat bradyarrhythmias?

Answers

1. This is a sinus bradycardia with a rate of 37 beats per minute (bpm). Assess using the ABCDE approach.
   - Give oxygen if appropriate and obtain intravenous access
   - Monitor ECG, blood pressure (BP), SpO_2 and record 12-lead ECG
   - Identify and treat reversible causes (e.g. electrolyte abnormalities)
   - If adverse features are present (shock, syncope, myocardial ischemia or heart failure) then treat with atropine 0.5 mg IV. This may be repeated to a maximum of 3 mg

2. Numerous surgical interventions can cause excessive vagal firing. These include:
   - Abdominal distension, for example during gas inflation for laparoscopy
   - Visceral retraction
   - Airway stimulation. May also occur during laryngoscopy
   - Extraocular muscle retraction

3. Risk factors for asytole include:
   - Recent asystole
   - Mobitz II AV block
   - Complete heart block with broad QRS
   - Ventricular pauses > 3 s

4. Additional methods can be pharmacological or nonpharmacological:

Pharmacological	Glycopyrrolate	IV bolus of 0.2–0.4 mg
	Epinephrine	IV infusion of 2–10 µg/min
	Isoproterenol	IV infusion of 5 µg/min
	Dopamine	IV infusion of 2–10 µg/kg/min

All infusion rates should be titrated to effect to avoid excessive tachycardia and hypertension. Glucagon may also be used in bradycardia secondary to beta-blocker overdose (adult dose is 1–5 mg IV with onset around one minute).

Nonpharmacological	Transcutaneous pacing using pads and defibrillator
	Transvenous pacing via pacing wires

Discussion

If pharmacological methods of resolving the bradyarrhythmia have failed, the interim measure of transcutaneous pacing may be required. Capture may be difficult and require 50–100 mA, the upper end of which is very uncomfortable for an awake patient. An anterior–posterior pad position may reduce the capture threshold in some circumstances. Judicious use of analgesia and sedation may be required while awaiting transvenous pacing.

2 Collapsed Obstetric Patient

Candidate's Instructions

A lady who is 36 weeks pregnant has collapsed in the delivery suite. Please assess and manage this patient.

Questions

1. Outline your management of the collapsed pregnant patient.
2. Why would you displace the uterus?
3. Which reversible causes of cardiovascular collapse are more likely in the pregnant woman?
4. What are the potential benefits of performing a perimortem cesarean section?

Answers

1. Approach rapidly. Look around to ensure the area is safe to approach and explain what you are doing as you progress.
   - Try and rouse the patient – if there is no response, **call for help!**
   - Head-tilt, chin-lift, look, listen and feel for breath sounds and a carotid pulse – if absent, start CPR and send your help to call the code team. This includes obstetric and pediatric code teams
   - Once you have a second pair of hands to assist you, place a wedge under the patient to give a 15 degree left lateral tilt. If there is no wedge present, use a rolled blanket or manually displace the uterus. Try and minimize interruptions to CPR
   - State you would perform early intubation with cricoid pressure due to the risks of aspiration in pregnant women. Say you would use a smaller endotracheal tube due to the airway edema associated with pregnancy
   - Once monitoring equipment is attached, perform defibrillation or administer drugs and fluid as per normal adult advanced cardiac life support (ACLS) guidelines. Remove all fetal monitoring probes and leads prior to defibrillation
   - Consider starting a perimortem cesarean section within four minutes, as it should be completed by five minutes
2. The gravid uterus can significantly compress the iliac and abdominal vessels, markedly reducing venous return from the lower limbs and subsequently reducing cardiac output.
3. Hypovolemia, thromboembolism and toxins are the most likely causes of cardiac arrest. Bleeding may be hidden, embolism may be caused by amniotic fluid, clot or air and toxins may be iatrogenic in nature (e.g. local anesthetic toxicity) or due to other pathology (e.g. sepsis, eclampsia).
4. Delivery of the fetus will negate the effects of aortocaval compression and improve the chances of successful resuscitation. It will reduce maternal oxygen consumption, increase venous return, make ventilation easier and allow CPR in the supine position.

Discussion

It is more than likely that a simulation woman will be used for this scenario. Do not be put off by the fact that the patient is pregnant, go through your ACLS algorithm as normal and remember the four key points discussed earlier. There are four additional requirements to resuscitating a pregnant patient:
- The code team should include obstetricians and pediatricians
- Left lateral tilt
- Chest compressions should be placed slightly higher on the sternum because the abdominal contents and the diaphragm are displaced cephalad during the third trimester of pregnancy
- Intravenous access should be obtained above the diaphragm
- Apply the same defibrillation energies as in nonpregnant patients, but remove all fetal monitoring probes and leads
- Early intubation, but consider airway edema associated with pregnancy
- Perimortem cesarean section

CPR should be performed in the same way and drugs should be administered at standard doses. Safe defibrillation may be assessed at this station so be prepared for the sequence of pulseless electrical activity (PEA) when you arrive (epinephrine but **not atropine**) deteriorating into ventricular fibrillation, which requires a shock. This may revert to PEA and you should be ready to commence the cesarean section by the second check, that is, at four minutes if there is no response to your resuscitation.

3 Malignant Hyperthermia

Candidate's Instructions

You have just taken over the anesthetic care of a 14-year-old girl on the plastics operating room schedule. The monitor alarm starts to sound. Her vital signs are given as follows:

Heart rate	129 bpm
Blood pressure	107/62 mmHg
SpO_2	92%
Temperature	38.40 °C
$ETCO_2$	68 mmHg

Questions

1. How would you manage this situation?
2. What are the features of malignant hyperthermia (MH)?
3. What are the risk factors for MH?
4. What follow-up is required for a patient suspected of having MH?

Answers

1. State that you think this is likely to be MH and proceed as follows.

   Immediate management:
   - Stop all potential triggers i.e. volatile agents and succinylcholine
   - Communicate. Alert the surgeon. Call for help and dantrolene
   - Install a clean breathing system and hyperventilate with 100% O_2 high flow
   - Maintain anesthesia with an intravenous agent
   - Abandon/finish surgery as soon as possible
   - Muscle relaxation with non-depolarizing neuromuscular blocking drug

   Monitoring and treatment:
   - Give dantrolene 2.5 mg/kg immediate IV bolus (repeat 1 mg/kg boluses as required to a maximum of 10 mg/kg)
   - Start active cooling
   - Place invasive arterial and central venous monitoring and catheterize if not done already
   - Take blood samples: arterial blood gas, electrolytes, complete blood count (CBC), coagulation studies, creatinine kinase levels, and lactate levels
   - Treat hyperkalemia with calcium chloride and glucose–insulin infusion, as required
   - Treat arrhythmias with amiodarone/magnesium/metoprolol. Avoid calcium channel blockers
   - Metabolic acidosis can be compensated for by hyperventilation and administration of sodium bicarbonate
   - Myoglobinemia may precipitate acute renal failure, the incidence of which may be reduced by inducing alkaline diuresis instituted by a combination of mannitol, furosemide and sodium bicarbonate with a goal of 1 mL/kg per hour of urine
   - Disseminated intravascular coagulopathy may ensue. Treat with fresh frozen plasma (FFP), platelets and cryoprecipitate as guided by thromboelastography or coagulation studies

2. The features of MH are related to muscle abnormality and hypermetabolism, but not all may be present:
   - Sustained jaw rigidity after succinylcholine (masseter spasm)
   - Unexplained tachycardia, rise in end-tidal (ET) CO_2 and oxygen requirement
   - Cardiovascular instability and dysrhythmias (especially ectopic ventricular beats and ventricular bigeminy)
   - Generalized rigidity
   - Rise in core body temperature by two degrees per hour
   - Metabolic acidosis

3. Risk factors for MH include a family history, previous exposure to succinylcholine or volatile agents (even if previous exposures were uneventful), central core disease (a rare disease affecting skeletal muscles) and King–Denborough syndrome (a congenital myopathy associated with susceptibility to malignant hyperthermia, skeletal abnormalities and dysmorphic features with characteristic facial appearance).

4. Follow-up:
   - Continue monitoring in intensive care; repeat dantrolene as necessary
   - Monitor for acute kidney injury and compartment syndrome
   - Follow creatinine kinase and urine myoglobin for 36 hours

- Consider alternative diagnoses (sepsis, pheochromocytomata, thyroid storm, myopathy)
- Counsel patient and family members
- Consider contacting the Malignant Hyperthermia Association of the United States (MHAUS), and arrange for family testing

Discussion

Do not rush into a diagnosis in this situation. Check and confirm readings as you would in real life and take steps to correct them as you find them. **Note**: a diagnosis of MH requires an unexplained increase in $ETCO_2$ with an unexplained increase in heart rate and an unexplained increase in core temperature.

These answers closely follow the malignant hyperthermia guidelines published by MHAUS, which are essential reading. MHAUS has four primary goals:
- Educate the entire spectrum of healthcare professionals so that MH is rapidly recognized and properly treated by persons in all of the medical disciplines
- Advise and prepare all medical facilities in the United States for prompt diagnosis and immediate treatment of an MH episode
- Help MH-susceptible patients and their families to learn to live with MH susceptibility and share with them the experience and knowledge which has accumulated about MH
- Encourage and support research in MH, especially a highly accurate noninvasive diagnostic test

It would not be unreasonable to ask how to mix up the dantrolene. Each 20 mg vial is mixed with 60 mL of sterile water, which is why it takes so long to draw up and administer. A typical 70-kg person will require nine vials (2.5 mg/kg) initially, and may require up to 35 vials (10 mg/kg) in total. A new formulation of dantrolene (Ryanodex) requires less water for mixing, but costs more.

4 Failed Intubation

Candidate's Instructions

You have just given the drugs for a rapid sequence intubation (RSI) on this patient about to undergo appendectomy. Please perform laryngoscopy and intubate this patient. You fail to intubate the mannequin. The patient starts to desaturate.

Questions

1. Describe the procedure for difficult laryngoscopy during an RSI.
2. If the patient is becoming hypoxic, without signs of spontaneous breathing, what steps would you take?

Answers

1. Ensure you have allowed sufficient time for the succinylcholine to work, that is, at least 45 seconds (some suggest one minute).
   - On finding difficult laryngoscopy, initially reposition the head, ensuring full neck flexion and head extension (sniffing the morning air)
   - External laryngeal manipulation with your free hand may bring the larynx into view
   - Consider asking for a transient reduction in cricoid force
   - Ask your assistant to apply backward, upward and pressure to the right on the thyroid cartilage (BURP maneuver)
   - A different laryngoscope or blade could be employed for a third and final attempt at laryngoscopy. Video laryngoscopy is also acceptable
   - If still unable to intubate, a failed intubation should be announced and the patient allowed to wake up while maintaining oxygenation

   Note: in the event of a failed intubation for an RSI in which surgery is not life-saving, the focus should be on maintaining oxygenation and waking the patient up, then deciding on another technique (usually awake fiber-optic intubation). The situation, however, is different for an RSI for true emergency surgery where the risks of using a supraglottic airway or other methods of intubation have to be balanced against the risks of postponing surgery.

2. Call for help and keep your trained assistant.
   - Continue to apply cricoid force at 30 N
   - Insert a Guedel airway and attempt facemask ventilation with 100 percent oxygen
   - If necessary, use both hands to hold the facemask and ask your assistant to squeeze the bag
   - If facemask ventilation is not possible, maintain cricoid pressure and insert the laryngeal mask airway (LMA). Release the cricoid pressure as you insert the LMA and reapply once it is seated in the correct position
   - Attempt to ventilate with 100 percent oxygen via the LMA with cricoid pressure
   - If this fails, release cricoid pressure and attempt ventilation again through the LMA
   - If at this point ventilation is still not possible and the patient is not waking up appropriately/unable to maintain adequate tidal volumes and their oxygen saturations are falling below 85 percent, you must declare a failed intubation, failed ventilation situation
   - Make sure help is at hand and proceed to a needle cricothyroidotomy or a surgical cricothyroidotomy

Discussion

This station is assessing your knowledge of the American Society of Anesthesiologists (ASA) practice guidelines for the management of a difficult airway. Do not get bogged down in the doses of anesthetic agents or what you use, keep it simple as time will be short. You will need to check all the appropriate equipment quickly and that monitoring is available and attached. In real life, a Peritraumatic Dissociative Experiences Questionnaire (PDEQ) check is invaluable:

Patient

- Positioned well on tilting trolley. Attached to cycling BP, oximeter, ECG monitoring, capnograph and 100 percent oxygen

Drugs

- Anesthetic and emergency (atropine, phenylephrine, epinephrine)

Equipment

- Different laryngoscope blades, scopes (fiber-optic, videolaryngoscope, etc.), various sizes of endotracheal tubes, bougie, suction, syringe and a tie. At the very least, you should have airway adjuncts and an LMA at hand and know where the cricothyroidotomy kit is located
- Refer to ASA difficult airway management guidelines

5 Displaced Tracheostomy

Candidate's Instructions

This patient has recently had a tracheostomy but is having difficulty breathing. The house officer has called you because he is very concerned and unsure what to do.

Note: check the instructions carefully for information regarding the type and reason for the tracheostomy placement as this may change your management. In particular, check if the patient has had a laryngectomy.

Questions

1. How would you assess a patient with a suspected partially displaced tracheostomy tube?
2. If a patient has had a laryngectomy, how would your immediate management differ?
3. What are the signs that a tracheostomy tube may be misplaced?
4. What are the recognized complications of a tracheostomy?

Answers

1. This is an emergency situation requiring both an anesthesiologist and ear nose and throat (ENT) support. The partially displaced tracheostomy tube is more dangerous than the one lying in the bed as it has the potential to be undiagnosed. Proceed as follows:
   - Call for help
   - Apply 100 percent oxygen to both face and tracheostomy tube
   - Inflate the tracheostomy cuff if it still appears to be in place and carefully assess breathing. Attaching a Mapleson C circuit with capnography will provide clear evidence of whether ventilation is taking place through the tracheostomy tube
   - Can a suction catheter be passed? If not, remove the inner tube and check whether it is blocked
   - If there is no improvement, deflate the cuff and check for signs of improved oral ventilation
   - If there is still no improvement, remove the tracheostomy tube, cover the stoma and attempt to ventilate orally, following the American Society of Anesthesiologists difficult airway algorithm
   - Note that this may require securing the airway by re-intubating orally
   - If a "cannot ventilate, cannot intubate" situation develops, return to the stoma and attempt to ventilate using a small mask or laryngeal mask airway
   - If this fails, attempt to intubate the stoma
2. A patient with a laryngectomy has no connection between their oropharynx and their trachea. Therefore, all attempts to ventilate or intubate the patient must focus on the stoma.
3. There are several "red flag" signs that may be suggestive of imminent displacement of a tracheostomy tube. Detection of any of these signs warrants investigation by an anesthesiologist. Red flags include:
   - Increasing ventilatory support or increasing oxygen requirements
   - Respiratory distress
   - The patient suddenly being able to talk (implying gas escaping proximally and the cuff no longer "sealing" the trachea)
   - Frequent requirement for (excessive) inflation of the cuff to prevent air leak
   - Pain at the tracheostomy site
   - Subcutaneous emphysema
   - The patient complaining that he/she cannot breathe or is having difficulties in breathing
   - A suction catheter not passing easily into the trachea
   - A changing, inadequate or absent capnograph trace
   - Suspicion of aspiration (feed aspirated on tracheal toilet – suggests that the cuff is not functioning adequately)
4. Complications can be divided into immediate, delayed and late:
   - *Immediate*
     - Hemorrhage (usually minor, can be severe if thyroid or blood vessels are damaged)
     - Misplacement of tube – within tissues around trachea or to main bronchus
     - Pneumothorax
     - Tube occlusion
     - Subcutaneous emphysema
     - Esophageal perforation

- *Delayed* (up to seven days post-procedure)
  - Tube blockage with secretions or blood
  - May be sudden or gradual and may occur at any time
  - Partial or complete tube displacement
  - Infection of the stoma site
  - Infection of the bronchial tree (pneumonia)
  - Ulceration, and/or necrosis of the trachea
  - Mucosal ulceration by tube migration (due to loose tapes or patient intervention)
  - Tracheoesophageal fistula formation

- *Late complications* (more than seven days)
  - Granulomata of the trachea may cause respiratory difficulty when the tracheostomy tube is removed
  - Tracheal dilation, stenosis, persistent sinus or collapse (tracheomalacia)
  - Scar formation requiring revision

Discussion

Like all emergencies, you need to inform the examiners that you have recognized this as a crisis situation and delegate someone to call for help. It is unlikely anyone will come and save you in the OSCE, so do not get upset when the examiner states that your colleague is busy in the operating room, etc. Do not panic if the tracheostomy tube is in the bed, follow the steps outlined earlier and apply 100 percent oxygen to both the face and stoma site.

Assess each airway in turn and check the adequacy of breathing. If the tracheostomy is less than ten days old, it is probably sensible to cover (use your hand if you have to) the stoma at first and focus on ventilating via the mouth using standard maneuvers and adjuncts. Be aware that if a "cannot intubate, cannot ventilate" situation arises, return your attention to the tracheostomy stoma and try to ventilate or even intubate the stoma.

6 Pediatric Emergency

Candidate's Instructions

You have been called to see a 5-year-old boy who was found unconscious by a nurse. Please assess him and proceed as necessary.

Questions

1. How would you assess an unconscious child?
2. How can you estimate a child's weight?
3. How do you calculate the defibrillation energy?
4. What are the doses of epinephrine and amiodarone and when are they given?
5. The child is hypothermic after resuscitation; what temperature would you aim for?

Answers

1. State you would first check the environment, to ensure it is safe to approach.
   - Check the child's responsiveness by gently stimulating the child and by shouting (do not shake infants or children with suspected cervical spine injuries)
   - If there is no response, shout for help
   - Follow an ABC (airway, breathing, circulation) approach
   - Turn the child onto his back and open the airway using head-tilt and chin-lift or jaw-thrust if required (be aware of the possibility of cervical spine injury and, if suspected, try to open the airway using chin-lift or jaw-thrust alone)
   - Keeping the airway open, look, listen, and feel for normal breathing by putting your face close to the child's face and looking along the chest
   - If the breathing is not normal or is absent, summon the pediatric code team at this stage
   - Remove any obvious airway obstruction and give five initial rescue breaths
   - Assess the child's circulation (signs of life) for a maximum of 10 seconds. Feel for a carotid pulse in children over one year of age, or a brachial pulse in infants and babies
   - If there are no signs of life, unless you are certain that you can feel a definite pulse of greater than 60 beats per minute (bpm) within 10 seconds, start chest compressions at a rate of 100–120 per minute in a ratio of 15 compressions to two breaths
   - Lone rescuers should perform about one minute of CPR before going to get help, unless the collapse was witnessed. In this case a primary cardiac event is more likely and defibrillation is likely to be needed

2. A rough and ready formula for estimating a child's weight is: (age + 4) × 2 kg.
   A Broselow® tape can also be used to estimate weight; although it may underestimate weights in obese children, it is probably more accurate than physician-orientated estimates.
   A more accurate way weight is calculated:

1–12 months	(0.5 × age in months) + 9
1–5 years	(2 × age in years) + 5
6–12 years	4 × age in years

   You may not be expected to know this but it would impress the examiner.

3. Defibrillation energy is 4 J/kg.

4. Epinephrine is given as soon as intravenous access is achieved in non-shockable rhythms and after the third shock in shockable rhythms. The dose is 10 µg/kg, which equates to 0.1 mL/kg of the standard 1:10,000 solution. Amiodarone is given with the epinephrine after the third shock at a dose of 5 mg/kg.

5. A child who regains a spontaneous circulation but remains comatose after cardiopulmonary arrest may benefit from being cooled to a core temperature of 32–34 °C for at least 24 hours. The successfully resuscitated child with hypothermia and return of spontaneous circulation should not be rewarmed actively unless the core temperature is below 32 °C. Following a period of mild hypothermia, rewarm the child slowly at 0.25–0.5 °C per hour.

Discussion

The pediatric choking algorithm may also be assessed. This can be summarized as follows:

- Encourage coughing; if effective, observe the child closely for any sign of deterioration
- If the cough is ineffective, give five back blows followed by five abdominal thrusts for a child over one year old and five chest thrusts if less than one year of age
- If the child becomes unconscious, open the airway and give five rescue breaths and continue the Pediatric Advanced Life Support (PALS) algorithm

The acronym "WETFLAG" has been coined for use in pediatric arrest situations:

Weight	(age + 4) × 2 or use the new formula
Epinephrine	10 µg/kg (0.1 mL/kg of 1:10,000)
Energy	4 J/kg for defibrillation
Tube	age/4 + 4 for endotracheal tube sizing
Fluid	20 mL/kg fluid bolus
Lorazepam	0.1 mg/kg
Amiodarone	5 mg/kg
Glucose	2 mL/kg of 10% dextrose

7 Intraoperative Desaturation

Candidate's Instructions

You are covering for a colleague and have taken over the anesthetic care of this patient undergoing a laparoscopic cholecystectomy. The patient is intubated. The monitor alarm begins to sound as the saturations read 90 percent. Please proceed as required.

Questions

1. How would you manage an acute desaturation during anesthesia?
2. What signs might you detect if the patient had developed acute bronchospasm?
3. How would you treat bronchospasm?
4. How would you treat suspected tension pneumothorax during anesthesia?
5. How may laparoscopic surgery predispose to hypoxia?

Answers

1. A suggested method of approaching this scenario is as follows:
   - Confirm the pulse oximeter is reading accurately and inform the operating room team and surgeons that this is a critical situation while calling for anesthesia help
   - Hand ventilate with 100 percent FiO_2 while watching and feeling for chest movement
   - Check the capnography trace
   - Begin a systematic ABC examination starting at the patient and working back to the machine
     - **Airway** – Check the position of the endotracheal tube (ETT) to ensure it has not been displaced; check patency with suction catheter; feel for compliance while hand ventilating
     - **Breathing** – Auscultate bilaterally; are there any signs of endobronchial intubation? Is chest expansion bilateral? Can you hear a wheeze or crackles?
     - **Circulation** – A poor oximetry trace may be the first sign of cardiovascular collapse
     - Confirm you have airflow and oxygen within the circuit and check the circuit for patency and leaks. If uncertain, switch to a Mapleson C circuit and alternative oxygen supply (you would need an alternative method of maintaining anesthesia in this case)
     - If there is no improvement, consider alternative causes such as a massive shunt or V/Q mismatch (e.g. secondary to pre-existing cardiac disease, developing aspiration pneumonitis, acute pulmonary edema, pneumothorax, etc.), poor oxygen delivery secondary to hypovolemia or thromboembolic disease, or increased demand secondary to sepsis or malignant hyperthermia

2. Acute bronchospasm manifests itself via increased airway pressures, a prolonged upsloping expiratory phase on the capnograph trace and expiratory wheeze on auscultation (absent if severe). Air-trapping and hyperexpansion may occur, which, in turn, can lead to reduced cardiac output and hypotension.

3. This is an anesthetic emergency requiring help and rapid treatment:
   - 100 percent inspired oxygen, warm humidified gases whenever possible
   - Increase the volatile concentration to deepen anesthesia and induce bronchodilation. Ketamine may produce similar results
   - A rapidly acting beta$_2$ agonist such as albuterol should be administered by metered dose inhaler (MDI) via the ETT with an adaptor. Eight to ten puffs of short-acting beta$_2$ agonist (SABA) therapy should be used since much of the medication will condense in the ETT
   - Intravenous terbutaline can be administered for refractory cases, bolus with 10 µg/kg IV over 10 minutes, then 0.1 to 10 µg/kg/minute; infusion may be increased by 0.1 to 1 µg/kg per minute every 30 minutes to a maximum of 5 µg/kg per minute. Side effects include tachycardia and dysrhythmias, hypotension, hyperglycemia, hypokalemia, and myocardial ischemia
   - Ipratropium bromide 250 to 500 µg by nebulizer or four to eight puffs, 18 µg/puff via MDI down the ETT
   - When compared with atropine (20 µg/kg IV), glycopyrrolate (3.2 µg/kg IV) produces bronchodilation of longer duration. Tachycardia may be a problem
   - Hydrocortisone 4 mg/kg IV (maximum 100 mg)

- Magnesium 40 mg/kg up to 2 g slow intravenous injection is used in status asthmaticus
- Epinephrine – For refractory bronchospasm, epinephrine in the operating room is usually given intravenously (IV bolus of 10 to 50 mg) or by continuous infusion via an infusion pump (2 to 10 μg per minute). Watch for tachycardia and hypertension
- Subsequent management will require arterial blood gas analysis, chest X-ray and transfer to the intensive care unit

4. Suspected tension pneumothorax requires immediate treatment via needle decompression using a large bore cannula placed in the second intercostal space, mid-clavicular line. This is a temporary measure and a chest tube should be inserted as soon as possible. Avoid the use of nitrous oxide and turn to 100% oxygen as soon as this is suspected

5. Laparoscopic surgery may give rise to hypoxia for two main reasons:
   - Raised intra-abdominal pressure can increase mean airway pressures, thus reducing tidal volume and minute ventilation, resulting in hypoventilation
   - Absorption of carbon dioxide may also occur. This effectively reduces the alveolar partial pressure of oxygen via the alveolar gas equation

8 Tachyarrhythmia

Candidate's Instructions

Please look at this rhythm strip.

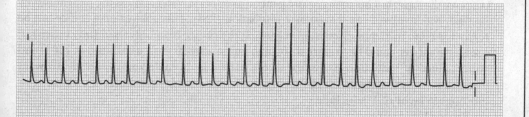

Questions

1. What signs or symptoms may suggest this patient is unstable?
2. How would you manage this patient if clinically unstable?
3. What ECG findings favor the diagnosis of ventricular tachycardia (VT)?
4. What is your first-line treatment for noncompromising VT?
5. How do you treat a stable and regular narrow complex tachycardia?
6. How do you treat a stable and irregular narrow complex tachycardia?

Answers

1. A patient with an unstable tachyarrhythmia may display the following adverse signs:
   - Hypotension
   - Reduced Glasgow coma score or syncope
   - Chest pain or evidence of myocardial ischemia
   - Signs of heart failure (cold periphery, clammy, breathless, etc.)
2. The treatment of choice for a compromising tachycardia is synchronized direct current (DC) cardioversion. This may require general anesthesia which, unless the patient is fully starved, will involve a rapid sequence intubation (RSI). This answer may suffice but be ready for more in-depth discussion regarding the choice of energy used (no consensus; a sensible answer could be to start at 50 J and increase by 50 J to a maximum of 150 J) and your method of induction. State that as the patient is unstable you would ideally want invasive blood-pressure (BP) monitoring although there may not be time for this.
3. Findings in favor of VT include:
   - Broad QRS complex
   - Marked left axis deviation
   - Fusion or capture beats
4. Amiodarone 300 mg IV over 20–60 minutes, then 900 mg over 24 hours (the latter needs to be given centrally).
5. First-line intervention involves vagal maneuvers (Valsalva maneuver or carotid sinus massage). If unsuccessful, adenosine 6 mg as a rapid intravenous bolus is given. If unsuccessful, give a further 12 mg and then another 12 mg while monitoring the ECG continuously.
6. Control rate with a beta-blocker or diltiazem. Consider digoxin or amiodarone if there is evidence of heart failure. It is likely that an irregular narrow complex tachycardia is atrial fibrillation (AF). The treatment for acute AF can become confusing when you bring in the need for anticoagulation and whether rate or rhythm control is required. As a general rule, if the patient is known to have chronic AF, then rate control will be the aim, with anticoagulation using aspirin if he/she is less than 65 years old and has no systemic disease, or warfarin for everyone else. New-onset AF requires optimization of any electrolyte disturbances, treatment of causative factors (e.g. chest infection, hyperthyroidism, etc.) and cardioversion, which can either be electrical or pharmacological. Anticoagulation is not required in acute AF if the onset is less than 48 hours previously.

Discussion

These questions are all based around the adult advanced cardiac life support (ACLS) tachycardia algorithm. Stations requiring a laminated ECG strip only are simple to set up. Make sure you can rapidly identify all the usual arrhythmias and can fly through the treatment algorithms without pause.

9 Anaphylaxis

Candidate's Instructions

You have just induced anesthesia and intubated a 19-year-old girl for a routine ear, nose and throat (ENT) procedure. The airway pressure alarm starts to sound. Her vital signs are:

Heart rate	132 bpm
Blood pressure	66/32 mmHg
SpO$_2$	92%
Temperature	36.4 °C

Questions

1. What are your differential diagnoses?
2. Outline your immediate management.
3. What are the early signs of anaphylaxis?
4. What follow-up will the patient need?
5. What is the pathophysiology of anaphylaxis?

Answers

1. Top of the list should be anaphylaxis! Others may be hypovolemia, endobronchial intubation, bronchospasm or an overzealous induction of anesthesia.

2. Use a stepwise and careful ABC (airway, breathing, circulation) approach:
   - Inform the surgeons if surgery has started and ask them to stop immediately
   - **Call for help** and note the time
   - Remove all potential causative agents and maintain anesthesia, if necessary, with an inhalational agent
   - Ventilate with 100 percent oxygen
   - Elevate the patient's legs if there is hypotension, whilst administering a fluid bolus
   - If appropriate, start cardiopulmonary resuscitation (CPR) immediately according to adult advanced cardiac life support (ACLS) guidelines
   - Give epinephrine intravenously
     - Adult dose: 50 µg (0.5 mL of 1:10,000 solution)
     - Child dose: 1.0 µg/kg (0.1 mL/kg of 1:100,000 solution)
   - If several doses of epinephrine are required, consider starting an intravenous infusion at a rate of 2 to 10 µg/min, preferably through a central line
   - Give saline 0.9 percent or lactated ringers quickly, through a large-bore intravenous cannula
   - Administer hydrocortisone 200 mg and diphenhydramine 25 to 50 mg intravenously Famotidine (H2 blocker) 20 mg IV may also be given
   - Take blood samples for mast cell tryptase as soon as possible
   - Observe the patient's vital signs over the next few minutes and reassess
   - If the situation is not improving, plan for transfer of the patient to the intensive care unit

3. The signs associated with anaphylaxis are not all present in every case. The majority of anaphylactic reactions include skin symptoms, which are noted in more than 80 percent of cases when carefully assessed; therefore, skin changes plus evidence of either respiratory compromise or hypotension makes the diagnosis of anaphylaxis highly likely. Other signs include bronchospasm, angio-edema and persistent abdominal symptoms such as cramp-like abdominal pain and vomiting.

4. Once the patient is stable, a further blood sample for mast cell tryptase is taken at 1–2 hours post-reaction. A third sample is taken 24 hours after the reaction. The anesthesiologist is responsible for ensuring that the reaction is investigated. The patient should be referred to a specialist allergy or immunology center. The patient, surgeon and primary care physician should be informed.

5. Anaphylaxis is a type I immune reaction, resulting from an antigen–antibody reaction on the surface of mast cells. Cross-linking of two immunoglobulin type E molecules by the antigen results in the release of histamine, serotonin and other vasoactive substances. True anaphylaxis requires previous exposure to the antigen responsible – anaphylactoid reactions do not, as they are most commonly due to direct histamine release from mast cells or complement activation rather than via cross-linking.

10 Obstetric Hemorrhage

Candidate's Instructions

You are in obstetrics half way through an elective cesarean section for which you have performed spinal anesthesia. Following delivery, the patient reports feeling faint and the obstetrician informs you there is significant blood loss.

Questions

1. How would you manage this situation?
2. Does the patient need endotracheal intubation?
3. What methods are available for stemming the blood loss in this situation?

Answers

1. As with all emergency situations, you cannot go wrong by saying you would call for help, declare it as an emergency and follow an ABC approach. Assess the patient quickly then initiate management, i.e. simultaneously diagnose and treat.
   - **Call for help** – get obstetric, anesthesia and operating room support
   - **Airway** – facemask oxygen, assess the airway, look for signs of obstruction and check the patient's conscious level if they are under spinal anesthesia
   - **Breathing** – look for tachypnea, labored breathing and signs of cyanosis and check the oxygen saturation
   - **Circulation** – look at heart rate, blood pressure, capillary refill time, peripheral temperature. Ensure you have at least two large-bore intravenous cannulae with fluid running through both and take blood for complete blood count, coagulation studies, fibrinogen, basic metabolic profile, glucose and cross-match
   - Quantify the blood loss (weigh the swabs if possible), ask if they have tried to stop the bleeding already, check the urine output
   - Get blood products urgently and designate one person to collect them. Most hospitals will have a number to call to initiate the massive transfusion protocol. Give O-negative blood if needed
   - If necessary, involve the blood bank's attending hematologist
   - Ensure normothermia by using a fluid warmer and active patient warming device
   - Request cell salvage
   - Talk to the patient and partner (if present) and explain all that is going on
   - Invasive arterial monitoring is useful in the context of ongoing blood loss and hemodynamic instability. Central venous access should be considered if vasopressors and care on high-dependency/intensive care units are to be considered
   - Administer packed red blood cells and fresh frozen plasma (FFP) in a ratio of 4:6, and give platelets if the level is $< 50 \times 10^9$. Cryoprecipitate should be administered if fibrinogen is < 100 mg/dL.

2. Indications for intubation include:
   - Reduced Glasgow coma score and obtunded respiration
   - Time following spinal anesthesia – will it still be effective?
   - Ongoing active bleeding and/or coagulopathy

3. It is always useful to know what the obstetricians are likely to want in this situation and pre-empt them, asking for certain drugs. Following are some options to consider.
   Pharmacological:
   - Oxytocin (Pitocin), IV: 10–40 units in 1 L normal saline or lactated Ringer's solution, IM: 10 units
   - Methylergonovine (Methergine), 0.2 mg IM injection (avoid if patient is hypertensive)
   - 15-methyl prostaglandin (PG) F2α (Carboprost, Hemabate), 0.25 mg by IM injection repeated at intervals of not less than 15 minutes to a maximum of 8 doses (contraindicated in women with asthma)
   - Some practitioners prefer direct injection of methylergonovine maleate and 15-methyl PGF2α into the uterine corpus
   - Misoprostol (Cytotec, PGE1) 1,000 μg rectally

- Recombinant factor VIIa is a treatment modality shown to be effective in controlling severe, life-threatening hemorrhage by acting on the extrinsic clotting pathway. Compared with other agents, factor VIIa is extremely expensive. Intravenous dosages vary by case and generally range from 50 to 100 µg/kg every two hours until hemostasis is achieved. Cessation of bleeding ranges from 10 minutes to 40 minutes after administration. Concern has been raised because of apparent risk of subsequent thromboembolic events following factor VIIa use

Surgical:
- Uterine massage
- Uterine packing – 4-inch gauze; can soak with 5,000 units of thrombin in 5 mL of sterile saline
- B-Lynch suture
- SOS Bakri tamponade balloon – Insert balloon; instill 300–500 mL of saline
- Foley catheter – Insert one or more bulbs; instill 60–80 mL of saline
- Uterine artery ligation – Bilateral; also can ligate utero-ovarian vessels
- Embolization of uterine vessels, requires interventional radiology
- Hysterectomy

Further Reading List

American Society of Anesthesiologists Task Force. Practice Guidelines for Management of the Difficult Airway: An updated report by the American Society of Anesthesiologists Task Force on management of the difficult airway. *Anesthesiology*, 2013; **118**: 251–270.

The following are useful organizations, including websites and guidelines:

Advanced Life Support Group, Managing Obstetric Emergencies and Trauma. See www.alsg.org/uk.

Advanced Life Support Group, Paediatric Advanced Life Support (PALS) resuscitation guidelines, 2010. See www.alsg.org/uk.

American College of Obstetricians and Gynecologists, Practice-Bulletin Postpartum-Hemorrhage, 2006.

American Heart Association Guidelines for Cardiopulmonary Resuscitation and Emergency Cardiovascular Care Science, 2010

Association of Anaethetists of Great Britain and Ireland. Malignant Hyperthermia Crisis Laminate, 2011.

Association of Anaethetists of Great Britain and Ireland. Management of a Patient with Suspected Anaphylaxis during Anaesthesia, 2009.

British Guideline on the Management of Asthma, a National Clinical Guideline No. 101, 2009.

Difficult Airway Society. DAS guidelines for management of unanticipated difficult intubation in adults 2015. See www.das.uk .com/guidelines/das_intubation_guidelines.

Malignant Hyperthermia Association of the United States. See www.mhaus.org.

National Heart, Lung and Blood Institute Asthma Guidelines.

National Tracheostomy Safety Project, www .tracheostomy.org.uk.

Resuscitation Council (UK), Adult Bradycardia Algorithm, 2010.

Resuscitation Council (UK), Adult Tachycardia Algorithm, 2010.

Royal College of Obstetricians and Gynaecologists Green-Top Guideline No. 52. Prevention and Management of Postpartum Haemorrhage, 2009.

1 Lumbar Puncture

Candidates' Instructions

Please describe how to perform a lumbar puncture (LP) on this mannequin.

Procedure

LP itself is not technically very difficult and by now you will have performed a number of spinal anesthetics. Anesthesiologists may be asked to perform the procedure when a neurologist is unable. Imagine doing the procedure while collecting your equipment and make every effort to ensure sterility where possible. The cleaning, draping and local infiltration should be second nature. The needle itself and the manometer may be less familiar. Make sure you have an assistant who can pass you pre-labelled sterile containers and a glucose bottle.

The pertinent points are outlined as follows:
- Obtain consent from the patient, explain the procedure and ask about any contraindications
- Assemble the appropriate equipment
- Position the patient – lateral or sitting
- Confirm your level by identifying for Tuffier's line at the level of L4 and identify a suitable level for the LP below this
- Indicate that this is a sterile technique and that you will wear a hat, mask, gown and gloves
- Clean and drape the area carefully
- Infiltrate the area with local anesthetic
- Insert the introducer (if present) and pass the spinal needle into the subarachnoid space
- Measure the opening pressure; note the color of the cerebrospinal fluid (CSF)
- Collect your samples in numbered bottles
- Remove the needle
- Cover with a sterile dressing

Questions

1. Where do the spinal cord and dural sac terminate?
2. What structures do you pass through with your needle?
3. What are the contraindications to performing an LP?
4. What are the potential complications?
5. Name three indications for an LP

Answers

1. The spinal cord ends at L1–L2 in adults, lower levels in children. The dura ends at S2.
2. In order, you will pass through:
   Skin → subcutaneous tissue → supraspinous ligament → interspinous ligament → ligamentum flavum → epidural space → dura and arachnoid mater → into the subarachnoid space.
3. Contraindications to performing an LP are:
   - Any cause of raised intracranial pressure
   - Patient refusal
   - Abnormal coagulation or thrombocytopenia
   - Local infection near the site of puncture
   - Congenital lesions in the lumbosacral region
4. Potential complications include:
   - Post-dural puncture headache. Incidence is approximately 1% with a 25-gauge, atraumatic needle. For diagnostic LP, a 22-gauge large needle is often used (for its higher flow rate), resulting in an incidence of around 25%
   - Infection, either localized abscess or meningitis
   - Nerve damage, which can be either temporary or permanent
   - Hematoma formation
   - Transient cranial nerve palsies (especially when large volumes of CSF are removed)
5. Indications for LP:
   - CSF analysis to aid disease diagnosis
   - Therapeutic relief of intracranial hypertension in benign intracranial hypertension
   - Intrathecal injection of contrast media and drugs

Discussion

This station may focus on either the explanation of the procedure to a patient (actor) or the demonstration of a practical skill on a model; therefore, you should be prepared to do both. What is required should be clear from the instructions and if you start asking the mannequin a detailed history about early morning headaches when you are being tested on the procedure itself, you will get a poor grade.

If the focus of this station is history taking and explanation to a patient, then knowledge of the disease states that may require LP is necessary. Some of these pathologies and pertinent questions are shown in the following table. After taking a brief history, it is most likely that you will need to explain how the procedure is performed and what information you hope to gain from it. Ensure that you seek cooperation from the patient and explain that you will stop if they are uncomfortable. This patient-centered approach is what you would do in reality and, hopefully, should get the examiner on your side.

Disease process	Specific questions
Subarachnoid hemorrhage	Headaches, visual disturbances, symptoms of meningism, vomiting, limb weakness
Demyelinating disorders	Visual disturbances, painful eye movement, ataxia
Benign intracranial hypertension	Visual disturbances, early morning headaches exacerbated by leaning forward or coughing
Viral or bacterial infections	Rashes, temperature, episodes of delirium

2 Chest Tube

Candidate's Instructions

Please describe how to insert a chest tube.

Procedure

Thus far in your career you may or may not have inserted a chest tube. Therefore, it is crucial that you at least demonstrate an understanding of how to perform the procedure. As long as you adopt a patient-centered, safe and aseptic approach you will do well. The key points are given as follows:

- Discuss the chest tube insertion with the patient, explain exactly what you intend to do and what position you require them to adopt
- Ensure patient compliance and understanding before going any further. Unless this is an emergency procedure, written informed consent is usually required, but this will depend on your hospital's policies
- You should ask for someone who is familiar with the procedure to assist you
- Proceed by collecting your equipment and positioning the patient appropriately
  - The most favored position is with the patient lying at a 45-degree angle with his/her arm placed behind the head
  - Some prefer to have the patient in a forward-leaning position with both arms raised and supported at clavicle height
- Employ a strictly aseptic technique – wash your hands and put on hat, mask, gown and gloves
- Prepare the skin with an appropriate (chlorhexidine) antiseptic solution and infiltrate in and around the insertion site with local anesthetic
- Insertion of a chest tube is normally performed in the "safe triangle."
- Make a 2–3-cm incision on the upper border of the rib, avoiding the neurovascular bundle associated with the rib above
- Bluntly dissect down to and through the pleura using a hemostat. A finger sweep inside the cavity ensures no lung is adherent to the pleura
- Inform the patient that he/she may experience some pushing and discomfort and smoothly advance the tube either in an apical direction, to drain air, or basally, to drain fluid
- Suture the tube to the chest wall (purse-string sutures are no longer advised), apply a secure dressing and attach the tube to an underwater drainage system
  Note that a Seldinger technique may be used with dilation with/without blunt dissection of the chest wall, particularly with smaller tubes, such as for Heimlich valves.

Questions

1. What are the landmarks of the "safe triangle"?
2. What are the indications for inserting a chest tube?
3. What are the potential complications?
4. Identify any errors or potential problems with this chest drainage system (expect to be shown photographs of incorrectly set up underwater drainage systems).

Answers

1. The "safe triangle" is the triangle formed by the anterior border of the latissimus dorsi, the lateral border of the pectoralis major muscle and a line superior to the horizontal level of the nipple (fifth intercostal space), with the apex in the axilla.
2. Indications for chest tube insertion are:
   - Pneumothorax in any ventilated patient
   - After initial needle relief of a tension pneumothorax
   - Persistent or recurrent pneumothorax after simple aspiration
   - Large secondary spontaneous pneumothorax in patients over 50 years of age
   - Malignant pleural effusion
   - Empyema and complicated parapneumonic pleural effusion
   - Traumatic hemopneumothorax
   - Perioperative – for example, thoracotomy, esophagectomy, cardiac surgery
3. Early complications include visceral injury, such as damage to the lung, liver or heart (and subsequent hemorrhage), injury to the intercostal neurovascular bundle and vagally mediated bradycardia.
   Late complications include post-expansion pulmonary edema, infection, aspiration of air or water into the chest, and drain blockage, which may result in surgical emphysema or even tension pneumothorax.
4. An underwater drainage system should exhibit certain features:
   - The drainage tube from the patient to the bottle must be wide with minimal resistance and have a volumetric capacity exceeding half the patient's maximal inspiratory volume to prevent water entering the chest
   - The end of this tube should sit 3–5 cm underwater
   - The bottle must remain at least 45 cm below the patient's chest
   - If suction is to be applied to the chest tube, it must be low pressure and high volume in character

Discussion

Any aspect of chest tube insertion may be assessed as well as knowledge of how to perform an emergency needle thoracocentesis. Consider dividing the procedure into pre-procedural considerations, performing the procedure itself, management of the patient with a chest tube and potential complications.

The explanation of any procedure starts with the patient and a discussion of what the procedure involves, why it is being performed and the associated risks. Once this is complete and any questions have been answered, the patient is in a position to give informed consent. Pre-medication with an anxiolytic and/or analgesic is recommended, as is a pre-drainage risk assessment, looking for coagulopathy or concerning lung anatomy, such as severe bullous disease. Imaging should be used wherever possible either to aid real-time placement of the chest tube or to mark the site of insertion prior to the procedure.

The choice of technique depends upon the size of the chest tube required. Small and medium chest tubes are most commonly inserted using a serial dilation/Seldinger technique whereas large tubes are only inserted by blunt dissection. Small-bore chest tubes are generally recommended for elective procedures, as they are better tolerated, whereas large-bore drains are recommended for acute hemothoraces, as they permit drainage of the thoracic cavity and assessment of continuing blood loss.

Patients with chest tubes should be managed only on specialist units by staff who are trained in chest tube management. A chest radiograph should be obtained after insertion. Bubbling chest tubes should never be clamped and there is no evidence to support clamping of chest tubes on removal.

3 Epidural

Candidate's Instructions

Please demonstrate how to perform an epidural on this mannequin.

Procedure

This station may focus either on the clinical assessment of a patient about to undergo an epidural insertion or on the practical aspects of performing an epidural on a model's spine. Be prepared to discuss both. Ascertain whether you are being asked to insert a lumbar or thoracic epidural; the procedure itself is exactly the same but considerations for thoracic epidural are slightly different.

Firstly, ensure the patient is appropriately prepared with a working intravenous large-bore cannula and full monitoring as per the American Society of Anesthesiologists (ASA) and American Society of Regional Anesthesia and Pain Medicine (ASRA) guidelines. Confirm they have consented to the procedure and are aware of what will be involved, then prepare and check your equipment. You should make sure that the local anesthetic is readily available and has been checked and that a working infusion pump is available.

- Prepare and check all your equipment and have a trained assistant at hand
- Position the patient appropriately (sitting or lateral) and check your level of insertion
- Use a sterile technique and put on hat, mask and gloves
- Check your equipment by flushing the catheter to ensure it is patent and assemble the Tuohy needle
- Clean the skin with an appropriate solution and drape the patient's back
  Note: concern has been raised over a possible link between using chlorhexidine 2% and arachnoiditis, so state you would follow local guidelines
- Infiltrate with local anesthetic at your chosen space
- You may choose to puncture the skin with a lancet to avoid pushing a skin plug into the tissue, and then advance your Tuohy needle into the interspinous ligament
- Attach your loss-of-resistance syringe and locate the epidural space using your chosen technique; for instance, constant/intermittent pressure with saline/air
- Explain to the examiner that you would warn the patient they may feel a tingling sensation in their back as you advance the catheter. Remember, if you are having problems threading the catheter **do not** pull the catheter back through the needle
- Once the catheter is in place, leave 4–5 cm of catheter in the epidural space
- State you would check for a falling meniscus, attempt to aspirate through the catheter and flush it to ensure its patency
- Secure the catheter with a dressing and connect it to the local anesthetic infusion
- It is advisable to give a test dose containing lidocaine with epinephrine to rule out intravascular or intrathecal placement of the catheter
- It is good practice to label the catheter as *epidural* and make sure everything is documented in the notes

Questions

1. What are the potential risks and complications of epidural analgesia?
2. Describe how you would check your epidural kit and prepare a patient for epidural insertion.
3. What are the features of a post-dural puncture headache?
4. What are the contents of the epidural space and what are its superior and inferior boundaries?
5. What level of block is desirable for an epidural used for labor analgesia?
6. What volume of 1:1,000 epinephrine must one add to 20 mL of 2% lidocaine to gain a final solution of 2% lidocaine + 1:200,000 epinephrine?

Answers

1. The approximate risks associated with epidurals are shown in the above table:

Complication	Likelihood	Approximate incidence
Hypotension	Occasional	1 in 50
Incomplete pain relief during labor.	Common	1 in 8
Insufficient block for cesarean section, therefore requiring general anesthetic	Sometimes	1 in 20
Dural puncture	Uncommon	1 in 100
Nerve damage	Temporary – rare	1 in 1,000
	Permanent (> 6 months) – rare	1 in 13,000
Epidural abscess	Very rare	1 in 50,000
Meningitis	Very rare	1 in 100,000
Epidural hematoma	Very rare	1 in 170,000
Accidental unconsciousness	Very rare	1 in 100,000
Severe injury, including paralysis	Extremely rare	1 in 250,000

2. The epidural pack should be sealed, in date, and contain a 16- or 18-gauge Tuohy needle with a Huber point. The catheter should be side-venting and should be flushed to ensure patency. A bacterial filter should be present as well as a clamp to attach the catheter to the filter.

3. The characteristic features of a post-dural puncture headache are:
   - Fronto-occipital headache that does not develop immediately but 24–48 hours after the procedure
   - The headache is worse in the upright position and eases when supine
   - Pressure over the abdomen with the woman in the upright position may give transient relief to the headache by raising intracranial pressure secondary to a rise in intra-abdominal pressure (Gutsche sign)
   - Other features that may be present include neck stiffness, photophobia, tinnitus, visual disturbances and, rarely, cranial nerve palsies

4. The epidural space contains epidural veins, epidural fat, spinal nerve roots and lymphatic vessels. The plexus of veins in the epidural space is called Batson's plexus. The epidural space is bounded by the foramen magnum superiorly and the sacrococcygeal membrane inferiorly.

5. A sensory block up to and above the T10 dermatome is required for epidural analgesia. Uterine and cervical sensory afferents are carried in the spinal nerves of T10–L1 and these are responsible for the pain associated with uterine contractions during the first stage of labor.
   The second stage of labor involves the vagina and pelvic outflow (S2–S4).
   The bladder, rectum and other pelvic viscera are also involved in pain associated with labor, and analgesia requires sensory blockade of L2–S5.

6. 0.1 mL of 1:1,000 epinephrine.

Discussion

In addition to the complications mentioned previously you may well be asked about some of the more notable procedural risks associated with epidural insertion. These are outlined as follows:

Bloody tap

Blood can be aspirated along the epidural catheter. Withdraw the catheter by 1 cm and repeat the aspiration. If blood flow ceases and an appropriate length of catheter remains in the space it can be used with caution. It is most likely that the procedure will need repeating.

High Block

The management of total spinal anesthesia may be assessed at an epidural station. Ensure help is called while cardiovascular and respiratory support is administered. A rapid sequence induction is required to ensure the patient's airway is secure and to allow ventilation. Recovery without adverse effects is usual if hypoxemia and hypotension are avoided.

Local Anesthetic Toxicity

Knowledge of how to manage local anesthetic toxicity is required and may also be assessed at this station. You should discuss the role of Intralipid following your assessment of airway, breathing and circulation. The current guidance is a bolus of 20% Intralipid at 1.5 mL/kg over one minute followed by an infusion of 0.25 mL/kg per minute. Further boluses may be given for asystole, and the infusion rate can be increased to 0.5 mL/kg per minute, but be sure that you are familiar with the latest guidelines for the use of Intralipid.

Subdural Catheters

A rare but documented complication (0.3–0.8%). Subdural catheters result in an uneven spread of local anesthetic, potentially producing a high block and Horner's syndrome.

4 Surgical Airway

Candidate's Instructions

Describe how to perform a cricothyroidotomy, demonstrating the procedure on this mannequin.

Procedure

Patient preparation for cricothyroidotomy involves neck extension and identification of the cricothyroid membrane, which spans the space between the thyroid cartilage superiorly and the cricoid cartilage inferiorly. The equipment required includes a cricothyroidotomy device, a method of ventilation appropriate for the device and a syringe filled with saline. Technically, it is a simple procedure, used either electively or in an emergency, and is outlined as follows:

- Obviously, if you were to perform a needle cricothyroidotomy for elective reasons you would explain the procedure to the patient and obtain consent
- Clean and drape the patient and stabilize the cricoid cartilage with the thumb and middle finger
- A 5-mL syringe containing 2–3 mL of saline is attached to the chosen device
- It is then inserted through the cricothyroid membrane in the midline, directed at 45 degrees in a caudal direction
- Gentle negative pressure is applied to the syringe, thus allowing the operator to see bubbles of air once the trachea is breached
- The cannula is passed over the needle into the trachea and air aspirated once again, to confirm its placement
- The device is finally connected to a suitable method of jet ventilation

Questions

1. What are the indications for cricothyroidotomy?
2. Why is the cricothyroid membrane used for transtracheal access?
3. What are the immediate complications of cricothyroidotomy?
4. What are potential late complications?
5. What favorable properties would you expect an emergency cricothyroidotomy device to exhibit?

Answers

1. Indications for cricothyroidotomy
   - As the final step during a "cannot intubate, cannot ventilate" scenario
   - Prophylactically, during an anticipated difficult airway
   - Electively, to provide oxygenation and ventilation by the subglottic route
2. The cricothyroid membrane is superficial (on average 8 mm from the skin) and lies 10 mm below the vocal cords. It is readily located in most patients by palpating a dip in the skin below the laryngeal prominence, is relatively avascular and does not calcify in the elderly.
3. Early complications:
   - Unsuccessful placement with the potential for catastrophic surgical emphysema, if high pressure ventilation is used
   - Bleeding
   - Posterior tracheal wall perforation and/or esophageal perforation
   - Pneumothorax and vocal-cord injury
4. Late complications:
   - Infection (and secondary bleeding)
   - Tracheoesophageal fistula
   - Changes to voice and subglottic/tracheal stenosis
5. Imagine having to use one of these objects in a real emergency and list the properties you hope it would exhibit:
   - Intuitive, easy to deploy with clear instructions
   - Safety features to help reduce damage to surrounding structures
   - A standard connector that allows you to attach the device to your anesthetic circuit
   - A long shelf life
   - A cuff and a diameter that allows both oxygenation and ventilation (4 mm or larger)

Discussion

Cricothyroidotomy devices are best classified according to their diameter because this factor determines the method of ventilation used and how the device operates. Small-needle devices (2–3 mm internal diameter), with a 13-gauge needle, are commonplace on most difficult-airway carts, but require a high pressure, such as that delivered by a jet ventilator. These devices will allow oxygenation but will not provide sustained and adequate ventilation. Needle-type devices require a patent upper airway, as exhalation is passive: if the upper airway is blocked, they can cause barotrauma. It is also worth noting that these devices have been associated with a high failure rate during the course of genuine emergencies.

Large-bore devices (4 mm internal diameter or larger) are used most commonly for emergency oxygenation and ventilation. These devices should be cuffed, to allow optimal ventilation. The last group of devices are those intended for insertion via a surgical technique and include endotracheal tubes (most commonly a size 6) and the Portex® cricothyroidotomy kit.

5 Central Venous Cannulation

Candidate's Instructions

Describe how you would perform central venous catheterization.

Procedure

This may require you to demonstrate the procedure on a model or may take the format of explaining the procedure to a patient who is about to undergo it themselves. You should be familiar with this procedure and, as such, only the salient points are highlighted here.

- Before starting, it is important to state that you would obtain the patient's consent beforehand, check clotting, review chest radiographs and rule out any contraindications
- Indicate that you would attach the standard American Society of Anesthesiologists (ASA) monitors and ask for a trained assistant and, ideally, intravenous access prior to starting the procedure
- Collect your equipment and position the patient appropriately
- State that you would use ultrasound guidance – as per ASA practice guidelines
- Wear hat and mask, wash your hands and put on your gown and gloves
- Open the central venous catheter kit with the help of your assistant, attach three-way stopcocks, flush all lumens of the central line and ensure you have everything that you require
- Prepare the chosen site with antiseptic solution, wait until it is dry and drape the patient. The drape should completely cover the patient from the top of the head to the toes
- Identify your chosen vein with ultrasound and infiltrate the area with local anesthetic
- Using ultrasound guidance, cannulate the vein with your needle, pass the guidewire, check placement with ultrasound before dilating, make a small skin incision and, having removed the needle, pass the dilator over the guidewire. Some centers first place a cannula into the vein and transduce, to ensure the pressures are venous and not arterial
- Ensure you always hold part of the guidewire and advance your line into the vein, aspirate all lumens, secure and apply a dressing
- Check placement with a chest X-ray if necessary and attach the central venous pressure transducer

Questions

1. What sites may be used for central venous catheterization?
2. Where should the tip of the catheter lie?
3. What complications are associated with central venous catheters?
4. What clinical features would suggest that an air embolism had occurred?
5. What is the landmark technique for internal jugular vein cannulation?
6. What are the relations of the internal jugular vein in the neck?

Answers

1. The most commonly used vein is the internal jugular vein as it is easily accessible, superficial in nature and associated with relatively few complications. The subclavian vein (higher incidence of pneumothorax) and femoral veins (higher incidence of thrombosis and infection) may also be used. Other possible sites include the antecubital, external jugular and axillary veins.
2. When cannulating the internal jugular vein, the catheter tip should lie in the superior vena cava above the pericardial reflection. If it is advanced further, the risk of arrhythmias, valvular damage and myocardial injury will be higher.
3. The complications of central line insertion can be divided into immediate and late complications:
   - Immediate – arterial puncture, arrhythmias (ensure ECG monitoring throughout), air embolism (reduced by head-down tilt), pneumothorax, malpositioning (e.g. internal jugular lines can go down subclavian veins and vice versa)
   - Late – vessel thrombosis, catheter-related infection, disconnection (may result in massive blood loss if not detected), migration and extravasation of infusions
4. Features suggestive of an air embolism include tachycardia, hypotension, chest pain, coughing, cyanosis, confusion, reduction in end-tidal CO_2 and tidal volume
5. The landmark technique has been superseded now by the use of ultrasound for all elective central venous catheterizations as per ASA practice guidelines. The landmark technique for catheterizing the internal jugular vein involves identifying the apex of the triangle formed by the two heads of the sternocleidomastoid muscle and the clavicle, inserting your needle at a 30-degree angle just below the apex, lateral to the carotid pulse and aiming for the ipsilateral nipple.
6. The internal jugular vein lies deep to the sternocleidomastoid muscle, and follows a course from the jugular foramen to behind the sternoclavicular joint, where it joins the subclavian vein. It lies alongside the carotid artery and vagus nerve within the carotid sheath. The vein is initially posterior to, then lateral to, and then anterolateral to the carotid artery during its course in the neck.

Discussion

The description of the technique you employ would vary according to the site of insertion. Most people will chose to describe an approach to the right internal jugular vein as it is likely to be the one they are most familiar with. You must state that you would use ultrasound guidance. If the examiners say it is not available then it would not be wise to proceed if the line is for elective reasons. In an emergency situation, and assuming that you had been appropriately trained, you could use the landmark technique.

Prevention of catheter-related infection is a topical area and, therefore, a question regarding steps to help avoid this complication is feasible. Considerations include:
- The choice of site – subclavian has the lowest infection rate
- Skin sterilization and preparation of the area
- Taking full aseptic precautions, including hat, mask, gown, gloves and a full drape of the patient

- The use of antimicrobial-coated lines
- Performing the procedure in a clean environment, such as in the operating room and not on the ward
- Ensuring adequate training of nursing staff and the use of an aseptic technique when the line is being accessed

6 Intraosseous Access

Candidates' Instructions

Describe how you would achieve intraosseous (IO) access in a patient.

Procedure

IO access is unlikely to be a procedure you have performed in anger but you may have practiced on a mannequin or chicken leg and, therefore, it should be relatively easy to explain. The advent of automatic IO devices may mean that this station focuses on the uses and management of IO access rather than purely performing the procedure.

The key steps in inserting an IO needle are:
- Obtain consent from the patient and collect your equipment
- Position a cushion under the knee, creating about 30 degrees of flexion, and locate the anteromedial surface of the proximal tibia
- Inspect the IO needle to ensure it is sterile and in date. Once opened, make sure there are no cracks in the plastic hub and that the trocar can be easily withdrawn and screwed in
- Clean the area and raise a bleb of local anesthetic at a point 2 cm below the tibial tuberosity
- Immobilize the limb and, with a screwing action, insert the device at 90 degrees to the skin until a loss of resistance is felt
- Remove the trocar, attach a 5-mL syringe and attempt aspiration of bone marrow
- Flush the cannula with saline, stating that you would observe for signs of subperiosteal placement or extravasation
- Secure the cannula with an appropriate dressing

Questions

1. When would you consider using this route for drug administration?
2. What are the recognized complications?
3. What are the contraindications to IO access?
4. What are the most commonly used sites for IO access?
5. How long should an IO device be left *in situ*?
6. What drugs can be administered via an IO device?

Answers

1. In adults, the use of IO access during cardiac arrest is becoming established as the route of choice if intravenous access is not possible or is associated with a delay in the first two minutes of resuscitation. In children, IO access is the recommended technique for circulatory access in cardiac arrest and is recommended in decompensated shock if vascular access is not rapidly achieved.

2. Complications include:
   - Difficulty in siting the cannula and subsequent failure to enter the bone marrow, which can lead to extravasation or subperiosteal infusion
   - Through-and-through penetration of the bone
   - Fracture or chipping of the bone during insertion
   - Local infection with the potential to develop into osteomyelitis
   - Epiphyseal plate injury
   - Skin necrosis
   - Compartment syndrome

3. Contraindications include a fracture in the bone proximal to the insertion site, signs of infection at the insertion site or an inability to locate landmarks (e.g. morbid obesity).

4. The three main sites for IO access are:
   - Proximal tibia (anteromedial surface, 2–3 cm below the tibial tuberosity)
   - Distal tibia (proximal to the medial malleolus)
   - Distal femur (midline, 2–3 cm above the external condyle)

   The army currently use a device called the FAST1® system. This is an IO device tipped with eight to ten needles introduced into the sternum in an emergency. It can be used to deliver any manner of fluids, including blood products.

5. The device should be used during emergency situations as a bridge until vascular access can be obtained. The manufacturers' recommended maximum length of time for all IO needles to stay *in situ* is 24 hours.

6. All standard drugs and blood products can be administered by this route. They should be used with 10 mL saline to ensure they reach the circulation, and infusions may have to be administered under pressure.

   Note: bretylium is the only drug that cannot be given via the IO route.

7 Anesthesia of the Eye

Candidate's Instructions
Describe how to perform a sub-Tenon block for a cataract operation.

Procedure
A sub-Tenon block is a popular block for ophthalmic surgery as it avoids the risk of needling the orbit. The Tenon's capsule is a white and avascular connective tissue layer surrounding the eye and extraocular muscles. As with all these stations, state that you would begin by explaining the procedure to the patient, obtain their consent and rule out any contra-indications. Then proceed as outlined below:

- Establish full monitoring, gain intravenous access and put the patient in a supine position
- Apply topical local anesthesia to the conjunctiva
- Clean the conjunctiva with sterile prep solution and then clean the surrounding area
- Retract the lower eyelid and ask the patient to look up and out
- Pick up the conjunctiva with a pair of non-toothed forceps in the inferonasal quadrant, 5–6 mm from the limbus
- Make a small incision using blunt-ended Westcott's spring scissors, which are passed inferonasally in a plane between the sclera and the Tenon's capsule. This will expose the white sclera below the Tenon's capsule
- Pass a blunt, curved needle (19 gauge) backwards beyond the equator and slowly inject 3–4 mL of local anesthetic
- There should be little resistance on injection and the solution should produce a slight proptosis of the orbit. Look for any signs of chemosis as you inject and stop if you meet significant resistance
- Remove the needle carefully and apply gentle pressure to the orbit for one to two minutes

It is likely that the discussion that follows will focus on the potential complications of ocular blocks and the advantages and disadvantages of the various techniques. There may also be a few questions on the anatomy of the orbit.

Questions
1. What are the most common complications of a sub-Tenon block?
2. What local anesthetic mixtures can be used?
3. Describe two other ocular blocks?
4. What complications are associated with these blocks?
5. What are the contraindications to peribulbar blocks?
6. What is the oculocardiac reflex?

Answers

1. Subconjunctival hemorrhage and subconjunctival edema (chemosis) are the most common problems associated with this block.
2. Lidocaine 2%, bupivacaine 0.5% or a combination of both can be used, depending on the desired onset and duration of the block. Hyaluronidase may be added to help increase the spread of the block but it has been associated with anaphylaxis.
3. *Retrobulbar block* – local anesthetic is injected into the retrobulbar space; this is the region located behind the globe of the eye within the muscular cone. This block is infrequently performed.
   Peribulbar block – local anesthetic is injected behind the globe of the eye outside the muscular cone but within the orbit. This is performed using a blind inferolateral injection (it may be supplemented with a medial canthus injection) of local anesthetic.
4. Retrobulbar and peribulbar blocks carry a higher rate of serious complications including:
   - Optic nerve damage
   - Globe perforation
   - Retrobulbar hemorrhage
   - Intra-arterial injection
   - Oculocardiac reflex
   - Subarachnoid injection
5. Contraindications to peribulbar block are:
   - International normalized ratio (INR) > 2.0
   - Axial length > 26 mm (increased risk of globe perforation)
   - Perforated or infected eye
   - Inability to lie flat and still – along with patient refusal, this is the only contraindication to a sub-Tenon approach
6. The oculocardiac reflex is a reflex arc triggered by traction of the extraocular muscles or pressure on the globe. This is sensed by the ophthalmic branch of the trigeminal nerve and relayed to the respiratory and vomiting centers and vagal nuclei. It can result in bradycardia, sinus arrest, respiratory arrest and vomiting. This is most commonly seen in pediatric strabismus correction surgery.

Discussion

The most commonly performed eye block is the sub-Tenon block due to its high level of safety. Describing one will be far easier if you have performed one yourself; try and at least practice one on a model before the examination. Questions may arise regarding the benefits of regional versus general anesthesia for eye surgery. Remember that most patients having eye surgery are elderly and are likely to have multiple comorbidities, making general anesthesia the more risky option. The problems with regional anesthesia are that full eye akinesia is not always obtained and, therefore, both a cooperative patient and, more importantly, a cooperative surgeon will be required.

8 Rapid Sequence Induction

Candidate's Instructions

Describe how you perform a rapid sequence induction (RSI) on this mannequin. Perform the procedure as you would in real life, stating which drugs and what doses you would use.

Procedure

The purpose of an RSI is to induce anesthesia and secure the airway in as short a time as is safe, thus limiting the time when aspiration of gastric contents could occur. You must stick to a logical sequence of events. The first and most crucial part of any RSI (apart from actually intubating) is the preparation. Tell the examiner exactly what you want as you would in real life. The checklist below may be useful.

Patient

- In a patient with bowel obstruction, consider placing a nasogastric tube to decrease gastric volume if this has not already been done, or measured by ultrasound
- Standard American Society of Anesthesiologists (ASA) monitors attached, noninvasive blood pressure (NIBP), ECG, pulse oximetry, capnography in the circuit that you will use to preoxygenate
- On a stretcher or operating room table that can rapidly be tilted head down
- Optimally positioned with cervical flexion and neck extension (as if trying to cross a finish line first – this has been found to produce better positioning results than the classic "sniffing-the-morning-air" position)

Drugs

- For an RSI, the usual combination would be induction with propofol and relaxation with succinylcholine; calculate the amount you are going to give in advance. The idea is that you can wake the patient in the event of being unable to intubate. A larger dose of rocuronium may be used, but caution is advised if difficult mask ventilation or intubation is anticipated. Rocuronium can also be rapidly reversed by sugammadex
- Emergency drugs must be ready too: phenylephrine, atropine and ephedrine
- Agents to maintain paralysis, hypnosis and analgesia after induction (these need to be ready before you start)

Equipment

- Circle system to preoxygenate
- Various face masks and airway adjuncts; beware of nasopharyngeal airways as they can (and do) lead to catastrophic epistaxis resulting in the loss of an airway in an obtunded patient
- Working suction under the pillow
- Various laryngoscopes of different sizes
- Endotracheal tubes of different sizes, checked, cut (if appropriate) and lubricated

- Bougie
- Tube tie
- Syringe to inflate cuff
- Suction catheters (paramount if airway soiling is anticipated, may be life-saving in bleeding tonsils where the trachea can fill with blood during induction)
- Rescue equipment to oxygenate in the event of failed intubation. Hopefully your preoxygenation will be sufficient to maintain the patient's saturations until he/she starts breathing; be prepared for this not being this case. A laryngeal mask airway should be visible; you should know where the cricothyroidotomy kit and emergency airway cart are located (and it should be nearby)

You need a trained assistant (or two) and a **strategy** for induction and intubation. This should consist of several plans and the team should be aware of what to do if one plan fails. Plan for failure.

Once you have everything in place (the hard bit), you can do the following (easy bit):

- Preoxygenate for a minimum of three minutes
- Administer the calculated doses of propofol and succinylcholine, 2 mg/kg and 1.5 mg/kg, respectively
- Apply cricoid pressure prior to loss of consciousness
- Wait for 45 seconds to one minute or until fasciculations have ceased
- Intubate
- Confirm the tube position with capnography, chest visualization and auscultation
- Release cricoid pressure
- Secure the tube in place

Do not rush this – there is a lot to remember. Have a logical sequence of checks in your mind and be clear on what drugs **you** would use (see failed intubation chapter).

Questions

1. How do you assess the airway preoperatively?
2. How can you assess the adequacy of your preoxygenation?
3. How is Sellick's maneuver performed?
4. How would you manage an episode of vomiting that occurred after delivery of the anesthetic but prior to securing the airway?

Answers

1. Airway assessment can be divided into history, examination and investigations. Elicit a history of:

   - Congenital airway difficulties (e.g. Pierre Robin, Down's syndromes, etc.)
   - Acquired disease (e.g. rheumatoid arthritis, ankylosing spondylitis, diabetes)
   - Iatrogenic problems (e.g. temporomandibular joint surgery, cervical fusion, oropharyngeal surgery or radiotherapy)
   - Problems documented on previous anesthetic records

   Look for:
   - Adverse anatomical features such as microstomia, large tongue, bull neck and morbid obesity
   - Mouth opening should be 3 cm or greater (measured between incisors). Less predicts difficult intubation
   - Mandible protrusion allowing lower incisors to pass anterior to upper incisors – Class A. Class B (incisors equal) and C (lower incisors unable to pass in front of upper) are associated with an increased risk of difficult intubation
   - Mallampati classification:
     I Faucial pillars, soft palate and uvula visible
     II Faucial pillars and soft palate visible – uvula tip masked by base of tongue
     III Soft palate only visible
     IV Soft palate not visible
   - Extension of upper cervical spine – a finger on the chin should be higher than a finger on the occiput at maximal extension (in the supine position). Level fingers mean moderate limitation; if the chin remains lower than the occiput, there is severe limitation to neck extension
   - Thyromental distance – the distance from the tip of the thyroid cartilage to the tip of the mandible, neck fully extended. Less than 6 cm predicts approximately 75% of difficult laryngoscopies

2. Adequacy of preoxygenation can be assessed by:
   - Measuring the end-tidal nitrogen level
   - Measuring the end-tidal oxygen concentration and ensuring a value of > 85%
   - Measuring the arterial blood gas and using the alveolar gas equation

3. The esophagus is occluded by extension of the neck and application of pressure over the cricoid cartilage against the body of the fifth cervical vertebra to obliterate the esophageal lumen. Pressure of 30 N (some articles suggest 20 N or even a range of 20–40 N) is applied before loss of consciousness by an assistant with thumb and finger either side of the cricoid cartilage. This is maintained until after intubation and cuff inflation.

4. If active vomiting occurs during an RSI, the cricoid pressure should be released, the patient placed in a left lateral, head-down position and the oropharynx cleared with suction. Active vomiting can only occur before muscle relaxation; therefore, there is only a small time window during an RSI where this situation may occur. Once the vomiting process has finished, reapply cricoid pressure, continue oxygenation until paralysis is established, then intubate with the patient in a head-down position (intubation may be attempted with the patient on his/her side but this may make laryngoscopy more difficult for the inexperienced). Failure to release the cricoid pressure during vomiting can result in esophageal rupture.

9 Transversus Abdominis Plane Block

Candidate's Instructions

Please look at this lateral abdominal wall and answer the questions below.

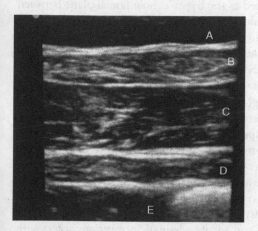

Questions

1. Identify the structures A to E
2. Identify the transversus abdominis plane (TAP)
3. Give three indications for a TAP block
4. What nerves are you aiming to block with a successful TAP block?
5. What anatomical landmarks would you use to position the ultrasound probe for a TAP block?
6. Briefly outline how you would perform an ultrasound-guided TAP block
7. What concentration and what dose of local anesthetic would you use?
8. What is the maximum safe dose of plain bupivicaine and bupivacaine with epinephrine?

Answers

1. A: Subcutaneous tissue
   B: External oblique muscle
   C: Internal oblique muscle
   D: Transversus abdominis muscle
   E: Peritoneal cavity
2. The transversus abdominis plane is identified as the hyper-echoic fascial plane between the internal oblique and the transversus abdominis muscles
3. Indications for a TAP block could include any of the following: renal transplant surgery, appendectomy, inguinal hernia repair, radical prostatectomy, cesarean section, hysterectomy and other surgical procedures involving the lower abdominal wall
4. The aim of a TAP block is to anesthetize the terminal branches of the anterior primary rami of T7 to T12 and L1 as they pass through the lateral abdominal wall, thus disrupting the cutaneous nerve supply to the lower lateral and anterior parts of the abdominal wall.
5. The landmarks are the costal cartilages superiorly with latissimus dorsi lying superolaterally; the iliac crest inferiorly, with the probe being positioned between the two in the mid-axillary line. This area is also known as the triangle of Petit.
6. In brief the procedure will include the following steps:
   - Gather all necessary equipment (20 mL syringes, local anesthetic, block needles, etc.), flush the syringes with chosen local anesthetic solution
   - Position the patient in a supine position and ensure adequate intravenous access with full monitoring, this should of course be already in place as most TAP blocks are performed under general anesthetic or following spinal anesthesia
   - Ensure a fully aseptic technique throughout the procedure
   - Identify the landmarks and place the ultrasound probe on the patient
   - With the probe and block needle held perpendicular to the patient the skin is punctured and the needle is identified passing through the subcutaneous tissue
   - The needle is then directed in a posterior and lateral fashion using an in-plane technique to visualize the needle throughout
   - Once the TAP is breached, local anesthetic is injected while aspirating every 5 mL, to produce an even spread throughout the TAP. This can be clearly demonstrated on ultrasound as a splitting of the fascial layers
7. Bupivacaine and levobupivacaine have been used in concentrations of 0.25% and 0.375% with volumes of up to 30 mL and 20 mL, respectively (weight dependent) for unilateral blocks. Alternatively 20–30 mL of 0.25% ropivacaine can be used, again according to patient weight.
8. The maximum safe dose of bupivacaine or levobupavicaine is the same for plain bupivacaine and bupivacaine with epinephrine – 2 mg/kg to a total maximum dose of 150 mg.
   Ropivacaine is dosed at 3.5 mg/kg to a total maximum dose of 250 mg

Further Reading List

Allman K, Wilson I. *Oxford Handbook of Anaesthesia*, 2nd edn. Oxford University Press, 2006.

American Society of Anesthesiologists Task Force on Central Venous Access Practice. Guidelines for Central Venous Access. A Report by the American Society of Anesthesiologists Task Force on Central Venous Access. *Anesthesiology*, 2012, **116**: 539–573.

Butterworth JF, IV, Mackey DC, Wasnick, JD. *Morgan & Mikhail's Clinical Anesthesiology*, 5th edn. McGraw-Hill, 2013.

Difficult Airway Society. Difficult airway society guidelines. See www.das.uk.com.

Gabbott D. Recent advances in airway technology. *Contin Educ Anaesth Crit Care Pain*, 2001, **1**: 76–80.

Graham AS, Ozment C, Tegtmeyer K, Lai S, Braner DAV. Central venous catheterization. *N Engl J Med*, 2007, **356**: e21.

Laws D, Neville E, Duffy J. BTS guidelines for the insertion of a chest drain. *Thorax*, 2003, **58**: S53–S59.

Longmore M, Wilkinson I, Turmezei T, Cheung CK. *Oxford Handbook of Clinical Medicine*, 7th edn. Oxford University Press, 2007.

Mendonca C, Balasubramanian S. *The Objective Structured Clinical Examination in Anaesthesia*. TFM Publishing, 2007.

NICE. Infection Control, Prevention of Healthcare – Associated Infection in Primary and Community Care. NICE Clinical Guideline CG2, June 2003.

Parness G, Underhill MB. Regional anaesthesia for intraocular surgery. *Contin Educ Anaesth Crit Care Pain*, 2005, **5**: 93–97.

Patel B, Frerk C. Large-bore cricothyriodotomy devices. *Contin Educ Anaesth Crit Care Pain*, 2008, **8**: 157–160.

Yentis S, Hirsch N, Smith G. *Anaesthesia and Intensive Care A–Z*. Elsevier, 2004.

Yentis S, May A, Malhotra S. *Analgesia, Anaesthesia and Pregnancy*, 2nd edn. Cambridge University Press, 2007.

1 Capnography

The ability to continuously measure end-tidal carbon dioxide (ETCO$_2$) is a relatively recent addition to the anesthesiologist's arsenal. First described in the 1940s, capnography has revolutionized anesthetic practice in the last 20–30 years. It can provide you with a multitude of clinical signs and is now part of the American Society of Anesthesiologists (ASA) guidelines for use in **all** situations where patients are anesthetized and intubated. You must know this topic inside out and back to front.

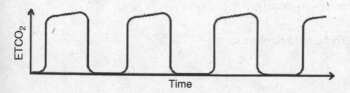

Questions

1. Look at this tracing and describe the different phases of a capnograph.
2. What is the difference in value between the ETCO$_2$ and arterial CO$_2$?
3. Give four examples of clinical information you can obtain from a capnograph.
4. What is a normal value for ETCO$_2$?
5. Draw the capnograph trace for:
   - Esophageal intubation
   - Malignant hyperthermia
6. Give three situations in which you would see a rise in ETCO$_2$.
7. What factors affect the measurement of ETCO$_2$?
8. What is the principle behind capnography?
9. What wavelength of light does CO$_2$ best absorb?
10. Give some characteristics of a sidestream capnograph.

Answers

1. Phases 0 to III:
   - 0 – Inspiration with sudden fall in measured CO_2 levels
   - I – Exhalation of dead-space gas
   - II – Exhalation of alveolar gas and dead-space gas with a sharp rise in CO_2
   - III – Expiratory plateau phase of mixed alveolar gas, peaking at the $ETCO_2$
2. In health, the $ETCO_2$ is typically 2–5 mmHg lower than the value for arterial PCO_2; the discrepancy is altered with V/Q mismatch and changes in physiologic dead space.
3. Capnography can be used to indicate: $ETCO_2$, respiratory rate, cardiac output state, airway obstruction, confirmation of tracheal intubation, circuit rebreathing, disconnection and hyper-/hypoventilation.
4. Normal $ETCO_2$ lies between 30–40 mmHg.

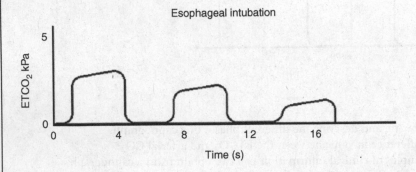

5.

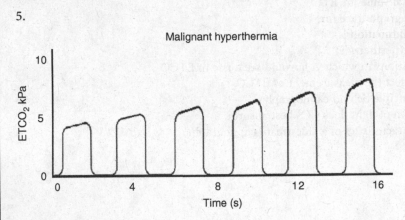

6. A rise in $ETCO_2$ may be seen with hypoventilation, malignant hyperthermia, sepsis, exhausted soda lime and laparoscopic surgery (CO_2 used for insufflation).
7. Nitrous oxide, water vapor and atmospheric pressure will affect measurement. Nitrous oxide absorbs infrared light in a spectrum partly overlapping that with CO_2. Collision broadening or pressure broadening is also a cause of error.
8. Capnographs employ the principles of infrared spectroscopy. Gases with molecules that contain at least two dissimilar atoms absorb radiation in the infrared region. At one end

of a chamber, infrared light is passed through a sample of gas – the greater the concentration of CO_2 present, the greater the amount of infrared light absorbed and the less is picked up by the detector at the opposite end. The signal is then processed to give an output reflecting the concentration of CO_2.

9. The wavelength best absorbed by CO_2 is at 4.3 μm.
10. Sidestream capnographs use a sampling line to draw gas at a rate of 150 mL/min from a connector at the patient's airway to an analyzer in the anesthesia machine. There is a moisture trap and an exhaust port to return the gas to the breathing circuit or to the scavenging system. They have a longer response time than mainstream capnographs.

Discussion

Capnography is a graphical representation of $ETCO_2$. Phases I–III represent expiration. Phase 0 marks the beginning of inspiration and a sudden fall in $ETCO_2$.

There is an initial flat baseline trace as dead-space gas that has not participated in gas exchange is exhaled; this is phase I. Phase II represents exhalation of dead-space mixed with alveolar gas. Phase III is the alveolar plateau, which usually has a positive gradient. This is a result of different alveolar time constants and the fact that poorly perfused and poorly ventilated alveoli with higher CO_2 concentrations empty later. The angle between phase II and III reflects the degree of V/Q mismatch present and may be substantial in those with respiratory disease.

Capnographs are highly informative and thus it is important to recognize set patterns. A sudden fall in $ETCO_2$ may represent cardiac arrest, air embolism or disconnection. Gradually rising baseline $ETCO_2$ may indicate rebreathing, soda lime exhaustion, poor gas flows or faulty expiratory valves. A slow rising phase II into III may be a result of airway obstruction or intrinsic lung pathology like chronic obstructive pulmonary disease (COPD).

Capnographs are the gold standard for confirming tracheal intubation. Increased $ETCO_2$ is seen in hypoventilation, sepsis, malignant hyperthermia, tourniquet release, increased cardiac output and bicarbonate infusion. Reduced $ETCO_2$ is seen in hyperventilation, bronchospasm, cardiac arrest, pulmonary emboli and hypothermia.

Two types of capnograph exist:
- *Mainstream* – Heated analyzers, sitting close to the airway. No sample line, rapid response time with no pollution and a less complex system. They are, however, bulky, fragile, expensive and may cause burns
- *Sidestream* – Most common type, away from the airway. Thin sample line with 50–250 mL/min flow rate, robust, less bulky. Transit time around 0.5–1 s, requires pump and water trap. Gases are returned to the circuit or out the back of the capnograph (hopefully to the scavenger system)

2 Central Venous Pressure Trace

When you are beeped at some unholy hour in the morning by one of your medical colleagues requesting your help with the insertion of a central line, you may curse yourself for choosing a career in anesthesia. However, as well as there being a strange satisfaction in seeing a text book central venous pressure (CVP) waveform from your expertly placed line, you can gain a great deal more information about the patient's clinical condition. This is what they will be testing you on in the OSCE.

Questions

1. Draw and label the CVP waveform
2. What do points a, c, x, v and y represent?
3. Between which points does ventricular systole occur?
4. What does CVP represent?
5. How is it measured and what is the normal value?
6. ˙What could cause an increase in CVP?
7. What changes in waveform would you see with tricuspid regurgitation?
8. Give two situations in which you would see abnormal 'a' waves
9. For what reasons might you insert a central venous catheter?
10. How do you differentiate between central venous pulsation and carotid pulsation?

Answers

1.

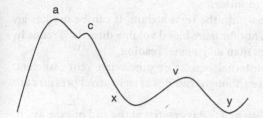

2. 'a' wave – atrial contraction
   'c' wave – back pressure against a closed tricuspid valve as the ventricle contracts
   'x' descent – atrial relaxation and downward movement of the heart during systole
   'v' wave – increase in pressure as the atrium fills against a closed tricuspid valve
   'y' descent – tricuspid valve opens, blood flows into the right ventricle
3. Ventricular systole occurs between the beginning of the 'c' wave and the end of the 'v' wave.
4. The CVP is the pressure present in the great veins of the thorax and reflects the pressure within the right atrium.
5. CVP is measured using a central venous catheter, usually placed into one of the large veins emptying into the superior vena cava. It is measured with the patient lying flat and the transducer at the level of the right atrium.
   Normal values are in the range of 0–6 mmHg.
6. An increase in CVP may be seen in: hypervolemia, raised intrathoracic pressure, cardiac tamponade, cardiac failure and superior vena cava obstruction.
7. Tricuspid regurgitation would produce so-called giant 'v' waves with loss of the 'x' descent and masking of 'c' waves.
8. Cannon 'a' waves may be seen in complete heart block; 'a' waves may be absent in atrial fibrillation, 'a' and 'c' waves may be indistinguishable in the presence of tachycardia.
9. Central venous catheters are used for:
   • Invasive monitoring of CVP – major surgery, shock, hypovolemia, intensive care
   • Administration of vasopressors, ionotropes, long-term antibiotics and drugs that are known to cause peripheral phlebitis, such as potassium chloride
   • Administration of fluid and blood products
   • Frequent blood sampling
   • In cases of extremely difficult peripheral intravenous access
   • Administration of parenteral nutrition
10. Differences between the carotid and central venous pulsation are:
    • The carotid artery can be palpated easily and is pulsatile with the heartbeat
    • The central venous pulse can be abolished when pressure is applied; the carotid pulse cannot
    • There are two components to the venous pulse; the carotid has only one
    • CVP can be augmented by position and the Valsalva maneuver
    • The central venous pulse can change with inspiration and expiration; the carotid pulse is constant

Discussion

Arrhythmias, changes in intrathoracic pressure and electrical interference will all alter the appearance of the pressure waveform on the monitor.

The CVP is used to indicate the pressure within the right atrium. It can be used as an estimate to right ventricular preload but does not measure blood volume directly. Trends in CVP may be more useful in guiding therapies than an isolated reading.

The CVP is commonly measured using internal jugular or subclavian vein catheters. It can also be measured using the femoral route although readings of right atrial pressure are less reliable.

In the healthy, spontaneously breathing patient, CVP is greatest at the end of expiration. In a patient who is being mechanically ventilated, it is greatest at the end of inspiration. The pressure should be measured at end-expiration, when the airway pressure is neutral to the atmosphere.

The CVP may be normal in left-sided heart failure as it predominantly reflects right-side function. Factors increasing CVP are given but CVP may or may not be reduced in hypovolemic states and with reduced intrathoracic pressure, such as with deep inspiration.

3 Electrocardiogram 1

Please look at this electrocardiogram (ECG).

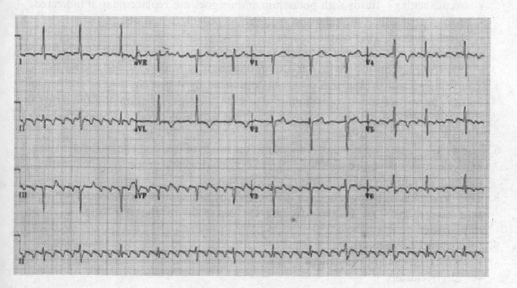

Questions

1. What is the rate?
2. What is the rhythm?
3. What is a normal P–R interval?
4. How would you manage this arrhythmia?
5. What does the ECG measure?
6. What is the frequency range for the ECG?
7. What are ECG electrodes composed of?
8. Why is this important?
9. What sources of ECG interference exist in the operating environment?
10. How do differential amplifiers work?
11. What is the common-mode rejection ratio?

Answers

1. The ventricular rate is around 80 beats per minute (bpm) with an atrial rate of 300 bpm.
2. This is atrial flutter with a variable atrioventricular block (3:1 and 4:1).
3. A normal P–R interval should be 0.12–0.20 seconds.
4. Options for managing atrial flutter include:
   - Acute setting – fluids with potassium and magnesium replacement, if indicated
   - Anti-arrhythmic – amiodarone, metoprolol, sotalol, flecainide
   - Direct current (DC) cardioversion
   - Catheter radiofrequency ablation
   - Anticoagulation prophylaxis is also important to consider
5. The ECG measures electrical potentials produced by depolarization of the myocardium. The bulkier the myocardium, the greater the depolarization and the larger the electrical potential detected at the skin surface by the electrodes. The normal signal value detected is 1–2 mV.
6. The ECG will pick up biological signals in the range of 0.5–100 Hz.
7. ECG electrodes usually consist of a silver/silver chloride electrode in contact with a gel medium containing chloride ions at the skin surface.
8. This arrangement helps to reduce interference by reducing polarization. Cleaning the skin beforehand and firmly adhering the electrode to the skin aims to reduce impedance.
9. Interference can arise from:
   - Shivering, patient movement
   - Electrocautery
   - 60 Hz electrical interference or noise
   - Capacitance effects
   - Inductance effects
10. Differential amplifiers amplify the difference in potential between two input signals, rather than amplifying each input signal individually.
    The benefit of using differential amplifiers is that any interference present in both input signals is nullified and the underlying potential being measured can be amplified preferentially.
11. The common-mode rejection ratio refers to the ability of a differential amplifier to reject the interference common to both inputs. A high common-mode rejection ratio is important where the signal of interest is of small voltage; for instance, most biological signals such as the ECG.

Discussion

ECGs can come up either in a physics-type station or a resuscitation scenario. Interpretation of the ECG will be expected in both. The station could cover a large number of topics, so be prepared for questions surrounding the configuration and composition of the electrodes, the electrical axis, frequency ranges of biological signals, amplifiers and electrical safety.

4 Electrocardiogram 2

Please look at the following ECG of Patient X.

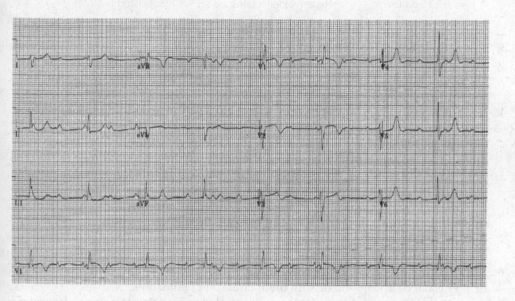

Questions

1. Is the axis normal?
2. What is the rate?
3. What is the rhythm?
4. Is it safe to give Patient X a general anesthetic?
5. Can this condition arise secondary to an acute myocardial infarction (MI)?
6. Given the rhythm, what signs and symptoms might Patient X present with?
7. How would you treat this arrhythmia acutely?
8. Is insertion of a pacemaker an appropriate management option?
9. Describe two other types of heartblock.
10. Give three considerations when anesthetizing a patient with a pacemaker for surgery.

Answers

1. The axis is normal.

Normal axis:	Leads I, II and III are all positive
Right-axis deviation:	Lead I will have a negative deflection, leads II and III will be positive with a greater positive deflection in lead III
Left-axis deviation:	Negative deflections are seen in leads III and II

2. The ventricular rate is 50 beats per minute (bpm) and the atrial rate is 100 bpm.
3. This is third-degree block or complete heartblock.
   Third-degree heart block is characterized by complete asynchrony between atrial and ventricular activity. There are no impulses transmitted from the atria to the ventricles, and thus an underlying ventricular "escape rhythm" is seen.
4. No. You would be very unwise to anesthetize such a patient and should seek cardiology advice with a view to management of the heartblock prior to surgery.
   Giving a general anesthetic with pre-existing third-degree block carries the risk of further bradycardia, profound hypotension and, potentially, asystole.
5. Yes. Acute MI is one of the main causes of complete heartblock, although usually transient. Other causes of complete heartblock include:
   - Coronary artery disease
   - Pharmacological – beta blockers, amiodarone, digoxin
   - Lyme disease
   - Congenital
6. Such a patient may present with collapse, dizziness, palpitations and shortness of breath or they could be asymptomatic with bradycardia on examination.
7. Acute management would involve increasing the heart rate using atropine or isoproterenol, external pacing (transcutaneous) and treatment of the underlying cause.
8. Yes. Complete heartblock is one of the indications for insertion of a permanent pacemaker. In patients unresponsive to pharmacological interventions, temporary pacing may be required prior to insertion. Other reasons for pacemaker insertion include:
   - Second-degree atrioventricular block with symptomatic bradycardia
   - Infranodal atrioventricular block, with left bundle branch block
   - Sinus node dysfunction
   - Post-MI – persistent second- or third-degree block
9. Other types of heartblock include:
   First-degree block: P–R internal > 0.20 seconds
   Second-degree block:
   1. Mobitz type I (Wenckebach phenomenon)
      Progressive lengthening of the P–R interval until there is a dropped QRS complex where there is failure to conduct an atrial impulse
   2. Mobitz type II
      Normal P–R interval with regular P waves but an occasional dropped QRS complex
   3. 2:1 or 3:1 block
      Varying patterns of P wave conduction so that the P wave to QRS complex ratio is greater than 1:1. These are described according to the number of P waves before each QRS complex; for example, 2:1 block is two P waves before each QRS complex

Mobitz type I is generally benign

Mobitz type II and 2:1 or 3:1 block can present with syncope and palpitations and can progress to complete heartblock.

10. Anesthetic considerations for a patient with a pacemaker are:
   - Ensure the pacemaker has been recently checked
   - Confirm the make and model of the pacemaker
   - Ascertain why the pacemaker was inserted
   - Use bipolar electrocautery in preference to unipolar
   - Electrocautery should be used as far away from the device as possible
   - There should be provision for temporary pacing, if needed
   - ECG monitoring must be clearly visible at all times
   - Have drugs such as atropine, glycopyrrolate and isoproterenol available

5 Humidity

While losing half your circulating volume, sweating in a heated operating room while caring for a burned patient, you may have wondered why it is so warm. Humidity is an easy topic to examine with important clinical applications and a wide variety of equipment you could be asked about.

Be sure to know the difference between absolute and relative humidity and that it is greatly affected by pressure and temperature. Appreciate its uses in anesthesia and have a good grasp of the various methods for measuring humidity.

Questions

1. Define absolute and relative humidity.
2. What are the units for absolute humidity?
3. What are the normal values for absolute humidity at room temperature, in the trachea and in the alveoli?
4. What is this apparatus and how does it work?

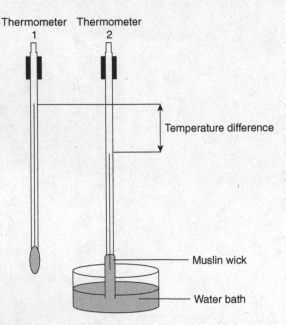

5. What other methods do you know of for measuring humidity?
6. What do you understand by the term "dew point"?
7. What is meant by latent heat?

8. What is meant by specific latent heat of vaporization?
9. Why do we humidify gases in anesthesia?
10. Describe three ways in which gases can be humidified.
11. How does a heat and moisture exchanger (HME) work?
12. Give some disadvantages of using water baths to humidify gases.

Answers

1. *Absolute humidity* – the mass of water vapor present in a given volume of gas at a given temperature and pressure.
   Relative humidity – the mass of water vapor present in a given volume of gas divided by the mass of water vapor required to fully saturate that volume of gas at the same temperature and pressure.
2. The units of absolute humidity are g/m^3 or mg/L (g/m^3 is used more often).
3. The normal values for absolute humidity are:

Room temperature (20 °C)	17 g/m^3
Upper trachea (34 °C)	34 g/m^3
Alveoli (37 °C)	44 g/m^3

4. The diagram shows a wet and dry bulb hygrometer.
   One mercury thermometer exists at ambient temperature and reads the true air temperature. The bulb of the other thermometer is surrounded by a wet wick; this thermometer reads a lower temperature due to the cooling effect exerted by the latent heat of vaporization. The rate of evaporation of water from the wick depends on the ambient humidity. The temperature difference between the two thermometers can be looked up in tables to obtain a predetermined value for relative humidity.
5. Humidity can be measured using a number of other techniques including:
   - Hair hygrometers
   - Regnault's hygrometer
   - Mass spectrometry
   - Humidity transducers – usually measuring changes in resistance or capacitance
   - Ultraviolet light absorption – uncommon
6. The dew point is the temperature at which the air is 100% saturated and, as such, water vapor condenses to form water droplets (dew).
   This is the basis upon which Regnault's hygrometer works and relative humidity can be calculated based on the dew point.
7. Latent heat is defined as:
   The amount of heat energy required to convert a substance from one physical phase to another without a change in temperature; for instance, solid to liquid, liquid to vapor. It is expressed in joules or calories.
8. The specific latent heat of vaporization is defined as:
   The amount of energy required to convert a given mass of liquid into vapor at a given temperature without a change in temperature. It is expressed in J/kg or cal/g.
9. Humidification is important in helping reduce heat loss and maintaining normothermia. It also provides a moist physiological surface for gas exchange at an alveolar level and helps with mucociliary clearance.
   The absence of humidified gases in the ventilated patient can lead to keratinization and ulceration of the airway, thicker secretions and mucous plugging, drying of the airway and poor ciliary function.

10. Methods of humidification include:
   - Water baths – cold or heated
   - Heat and moisture exchangers
   - Heated nebulizers
   - Ultrasonic nebulizers
11. An HME uses the principles of latent heat. The most common types consist of a paper or sponge gauze coated in a hygroscopic gel, such as lithium chloride. As warm expired gases pass over the HME, water vapor condenses and the element is heated by the latent heat of condensation. During inspiration, the gases are warmed and humidified as they pass over the now moist and warm filter.
12. Water baths can be simple cold water baths or more sophisticated hot water baths. Cold water baths are cheap but not very efficient. Hot water baths run the risk of infections, burns to the patient's airway, excessive moisture in the airway, and electronic malfunction and overheating. They can both lead to water gathering in airway circuits and thus affect ventilation, if present in sufficient amounts.

Discussion

As anesthesiologists, we should be concerned about humidity when ventilating patients, particularly in the long term. Humidifying gases aids gas exchange, protects respiratory mucosa, reduces viscosity of secretions and helps maintain normothermia.

It is also important to consider the humidity of the operating environment. Traditionally, the relative humidity of the operating room is kept at around 50 percent; this helps reduce the build-up of static electricity and minimizes the risk of fires and explosions. In addition, consider the environment in a pediatric or burn patient operating room, where temperature and relative humidity is higher in order to protect patients from excessive heat loss during surgery.

You should be aware of the values for absolute humidity in the trachea and alveoli and be able to describe most of the methods available for measuring humidity:

- Hair hygrometers rely on the fact that, as humidity increases, the hair lengthens and moves a pointer displayed on a scale to indicate the relative humidity
- Regnault's hygrometer consists of a silver or foil-wrapped tube containing ether. Air is bubbled through the ether until water droplets start to condense on the outside of the tube. This is the dew point and is discussed previously
- Exposure to water vapor in the atmosphere will produce a measurable change in the resistance or capacitance of a substance. This is the principle on which humidity transducers operate and are used to measure absolute humidity
- Mass spectrometry and absorption of ultraviolet light are other methods that can be employed

6 Invasive Blood Pressure

Historically, it is reported that in 1733 a priest named Stephen Hales first measured arterial blood pressure (BP) by cannulating the carotid artery of a horse with a glass tube. As you may expect, it did not end so well for the horse.

Having seen and presumably performed arterial line insertion (on humans), you should be aware of the various indications for invasive BP monitoring. The examiner may ask you how to perform the procedure but is more likely to question you on the physical principles surrounding the set-up of the system.

Try and have Laplace's law and the Hagen–Poiseuille equation in the back of your mind.

Questions

1. Give three indications for invasive BP monitoring.
2. What should the pressure in the bag of saline be and at what rate does it flush the system?
3. What are the required physical properties of such a system for optimal accuracy?
4. What information can you get from an arterial waveform?
5. What do you mean by damping?
6. What is optimal damping?
7. What do you understand by resonance?
8. Draw an under-damped and over-damped arterial trace.
9. What is the function of the transducer? Give an example of a type of transducer.
10. What are the disadvantages of invasive monitoring?
11. What factors affect laminar flow through a tube?

Answers

1. Indications for arterial line placement include:
   - Current or predicted cardiovascular instability
   - Blood pressure and arterial gas monitoring in the operating room or intensive care setting
   - Situations where noninvasive methods are likely to be inaccurate, like morbid obesity
2. The pressure in the bag should be well above systolic BP; usually, this is set around 300 mmHg, with a flow rate through the system of 4 mL/hr.
3. The ideal physical properties of such a system are:
   - Tubing that is noncompliant, as short as possible and with few interruptions to flow; for instance, a limited number of three-way stopcocks and connections
   - The arterial cannula should be short, noncompliant and wide
   - There should be no air bubbles in the system or clots at the end of the arterial cannula
   - The fluid used should be at a certain pressure and flow rate
   - The resonant frequency of the system should be without the natural frequency of the arterial pressure waveform
4. An arterial trace gives information about systolic and diastolic pressure, mean arterial pressure, heart rate, cardiac output and contractility.
   The position of the dicrotic notch and the rate of diastolic decay can also indicate hypovolemia and systemic vascular resistance, respectively.
5. Damping is a reduction in the amplitude of oscillations in a resonant system, due to the dissipation of stored energy to its surroundings.
6. Optimal damping refers to the ability of a system to respond rapidly to changes in the input value without producing excessive oscillations.
   The damping coefficient for optimal damping lies in the range 0.6–0.7; usually quoted as 0.64.
7. Resonance is the tendency of a system to oscillate at a greater amplitude when subjected to an external force, with an oscillating frequency close to its own natural frequency, i.e. when the frequency of the energy input matches the frequency of the receiving system.
8.

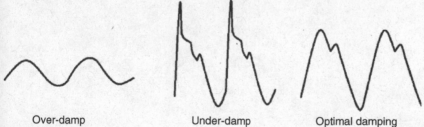

Over-damp   Under-damp   Optimal damping

9. A transducer converts one form of energy to another; in this case, it converts kinetic energy to electrical energy.
   Types of transducer include strain gauges, pressure transducers and piezoelectric transducers.

10. Disadvantages are: risk of infection, arterial damage (increased with multiple attempts at cannulation), peripheral ischemia, thrombi, errors in the measuring system and potential for hemorrhage.

11. Factors affecting laminar flow are given in the Hagen–Poiseuille equation; they are:

  - Pressure gradient ΔP
  - Radius or diameter
  - Viscosity of fluid
  - Length of the tube

$Q = \frac{\Delta p \Pi r^4}{8 \mu l}$, where Q is flow, Δp is the pressure difference, r is radius, μ is dynamic viscosity, l is length, Π is 3.14 . . .

7 Respiratory 1

Questions

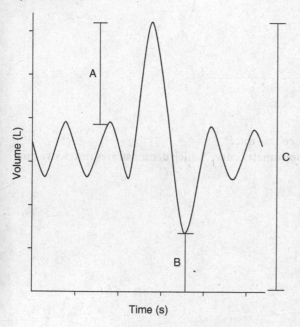

1. Label and give normal values for A, B and C above.
2. What is functional residual capacity (FRC)?
3. What can cause a fall in FRC?
4. Define FEV_1.
5. Define FVC.
6. What is a normal FEV_1: FVC ratio?
7. What pattern of lung disease does this spirometry trace represent? Why?

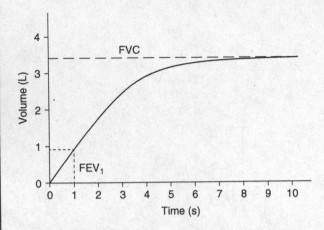

8. What disease processes may produce this trace?
9. What might you expect to see in a spirometry curve, which demonstrates restrictive lung disease?

Answers

1.

A = inspiratory reserve volume	2,500 mL
B = residual volume	1,500 mL
C = total lung capacity	6,000 mL

2. FRC is the volume of air present in the lungs at the end of normal expiration. It is a combination of residual volume and expiratory reserve volume. It usually measures around 2500–3000 mL.

3. Causes of reduced FRC include:
   - General anesthesia
   - Obesity
   - Lying supine
   - Restrictive lung disease. It is a common misconception that the FRC changes with age. It does not!

4. FEV_1, the forced expiratory volume in 1 s, is the volume of air forcefully exhaled in one second.

5. FVC, the forced vital capacity, is the maximum volume of air that can be forcefully exhaled in one breath.

6. The normal FEV_1:FVC ratio is 75–80%.

7. This shows obstructive lung disease.
   The FEV_1 is much lower than normal, being around 1 L, while the FVC is preserved, and the FEV_1:FVC ratio is therefore also markedly lower at 30%. This shows significant obstructive airways disease.

8. Obstructive airways pathology is most commonly seen in asthma, emphysema and chronic bronchitis. Chronic obstructive pulmonary disease (COPD) is a disease process encompassing both emphysema and chronic bronchitis.

9. A vitalograph trace of restrictive lung disease would illustrate both reduced FEV_1 and FVC, the FVC being more affected than the FEV_1. Thus, the FEV_1: FVC ratio is either normal or greater than normal.

8 Respiratory 2

Questions

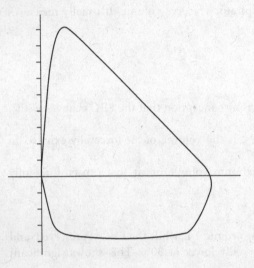

1. Label the axis in the diagram and provide values for the Y-axis.
2. Indicate which curve represents inspiration and which represents expiration.
3. Is this a normal flow volume loop?
4. Draw flow volume loops for restrictive and obstructive airways pathologies.
5. What pathologies do the following flow–volume loops represent?

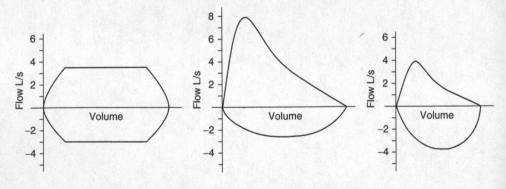

6. What is peak expiratory flow rate? State some normal values.
7. What two factors determine peak expiratory flow rate (PEFR) in health?
8. What is compliance and what are its units of measurement?
9. What factors may decrease or increase lung compliance?
10. Draw a pressure–volume curve for normal respiration.

Answers

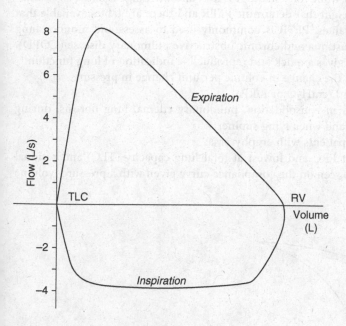

1. The X-axis is volume in liters.
   The Y-axis is flow in liters per second; values typically range from −8 to +8 L/s.
2. The curve below the X-axis is inspiration, i.e. negative flow, and the curve above the X-axis represents expiration.
3. This represents a normal flow volume loop with an absence of lung disease.
4.

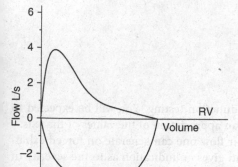

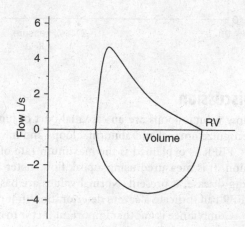

A. *Obstructive pattern*   B. *Restrictive pattern*

5. From left to right they represent fixed airway obstruction, extrathoracic airway obstruction and intrathoracic airway obstruction.

6. Peak expiratory flow rate is a patient's maximum rate of exhalation. Typical values for males are 450–600 L/min while for females it is less, and the range is 300–500 L/min.

7. In health, it is age and height that determine PEFR and there are tables available that show the full range of values. PEFR is commonly used to assess and monitor lung function in people with asthma and chronic obstructive pulmonary disease (COPD). It is easy to perform and gives a quick and reproducible indication of lung function.

8. Compliance is defined as the change in volume per unit change in pressure. It is measured either in mL/cmH$_2$O or L/kPa.

9. Compliance is decreased in consolidation, pulmonary edema, lung fibrosis, during laparoscopic procedures and when lying supine.
   Compliance is higher in patients with emphysema.
   Compliance is highest at FRC and lowest at total lung capacity (TLC) and residual volume (RV); this can be seen on the compliance curve given with a pressure–volume graph.

10.

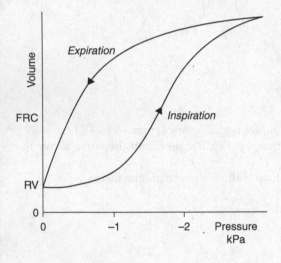

Discussion

Flow volume loops are an essential part of lung function testing. You will be expected to recognize normal and abnormal loops and have an appreciation of the values of the axis.

PEFR as explained is the maximum rate of air flow one can generate on forced exhalation. It is measured using a peak flow meter and gives an indication as to the severity of lung disease, if present. Normal values are based on age and height. A significant drop in PEFR can indicate a severe deterioration in lung function.

Compliance is another important factor to consider when assessing lung function. Total thoracic compliance takes into account lung compliance and chest wall compliance.

Normal lung compliance is around 200 mL/cmH$_2$O. It is increased in emphysema and decreased in infection, pulmonary edema, fibrosis and when lying supine (secondary to a reduced FRC). Lung compliance can also be described as either dynamic or static. Static compliance is the change in volume per given change in pressure during a steady state.

Dynamic lung compliance is the change in volume per unit change in pressure measured during air movement.

Chest-wall compliance essentially refers to the ability of the rib cage and musculature to expand and recoil. Chest-wall compliance can be reduced in kyphosis, obesity and circumferential burns to the thorax (hence the need for escharotomies). However, it is difficult to quantify and measure.

It is also important to appreciate that lung compliance varies with inspiration and expiration; it therefore displays *hysteresis*. This phenomenon can be demonstrated in the pressure–volume graphs that give a so-called "compliance curve."

9 Noninvasive Blood Pressure

The history here is a little less exciting than that of invasive blood pressure (BP) monitoring. However, you might impress the examiner if you tell them that the well-known Heinrich von Recklinghausen was a German scientist born in 1867 and his oscillotonometer was the first BP monitor that did not require the use of a stethoscope. They may then ask you about it.

On a more serious note, the advent of automated BP monitoring has permitted safer practice throughout the medical profession. There are a variety of noninvasive blood pressure (NIBP) measuring techniques available but not all are in everyday use. You are likely to be asked about the more common ones, the principles on which they are based and their limitations.

Questions

1. What is mean arterial pressure and how is it calculated?
2. What indirect methods of measuring BP do you know?
3. What are Korotkoff sounds?
4. What is the principle of the Penaz technique?
5. What are the disadvantages of oscillometry?
6. What problems occur if the cuff width is incorrect?
7. How do you size an NIBP cuff?
8. What sources of error exist with indirect measuring techniques?
9. Which nerves are vulnerable to damage by NIBP cuffs?
10. What is the suggested minimum inflation interval? Why is this?

Answers

1. Mean arterial pressure is the average arterial BP over the course of one cardiac cycle. It is commonly calculated as follows:

   Diastolic pressure + 1/3 (systolic pressure – diastolic pressure). Invasive monitors integrate the area under the curve and divide by the cycle time.

2. BP can be measured indirectly by means of:
   - Sphygmomanometer and stethoscope
   - Von Recklinghausen's oscillotonometer
   - Penaz technique
   - Oscillometry
   - Doppler ultrasound

3. Korotkoff sounds are heard while auscultating over the brachial artery when using a sphygmomanometer to measure BP indirectly. Nikolai Korotkoff described five sounds:

   I Repetitive tapping, synchronous with pulse, representing systolic pressure
   II Softer sounds, heard just below systolic pressure
   III Louder tapping sound as you approach diastolic pressure
   IV Muffled or muted sounds, within 10 mmHg of diastolic pressure
   V The disappearance of sounds, said to be diastolic pressure

4. The Penaz technique gives a continuous NIBP reading by sensing the volume of blood present in the digital arteries as it varies during the cardiac cycle. It consists of a small cuff placed over the distal portion of the finger and employs an infrared beam in combination with a servo-control valve. Together with a transducer, this apparatus provides a continuous tracing of the pressure in the digital artery as it dilates in systole and contracts in diastole.

5. Disadvantages of oscillometry are:
   - Less reliable in the presence of arrhythmias
   - Accuracy varies at the extremes of BP; they under-read at high pressures and over-read at low pressure
   - Pain and discomfort
   - Nerve injury
   - Tissue ischemia and skin tears have been reported during use in long procedures and in the elderly

6. If a cuff is too wide, it can under-read the BP or not record it. If the cuff is too narrow, it can over-read BP or not record it.

7. Cuffs are sized on the diameter of the midpoint of the upper arm and come in sizes from neonate up to extra-large adult. Adult cuffs should cover around two-thirds of the upper arm in length or be 20 percent greater in width than the upper-arm diameter.

8. Errors can occur with: incorrect cuff size, damaged leads, cuff leaks, calibration drift and variable ability to detect Korotkoff sounds.

9. The radial and ulnar nerves are the most commonly injured nerves. This can occur with prolonged and increased frequency of NIBP measurements.

10. The inflation interval ideally should not be less than two minutes. Shorter intervals between inflation cycles can give inaccurate results, lead to venous congestion, tissue ischemia and nerve damage.

Discussion

Modern-day techniques of measuring BP noninvasively tend to use the principle of oscill-ometry. One example of a device using this method is the DINAMAP, which stands for "device for indirect noninvasive automated mean arterial pressure."

The cuff is placed over the artery and inflated to a pressure above that of the previous systolic pressure. A release valve incrementally deflates the cuff. The unit combines a microprocessor and pressure transducer that senses the oscillations produced. The largest oscillations for the lowest pressure is the mean arterial pressure (MAP). These devices are said to be accurate to +/−2%.

Von Recklinghausen's oscillotonometer, although now obsolete, may be asked about. It employed two different sizes of cuff, one large cuff overlapping a smaller one. As the cuffs were inflated and subsequently deflated, oscillations produced by the pulsatile artery were detected via a needle on a pressure gauge. Systolic BP was marked as the oscillations first appeared and diastolic pressure as they disappeared. The smaller cuff permitted detection of the oscillations at lower pressures as the larger cuff was deflated.

10 Oxygen Measurement 1

Questions

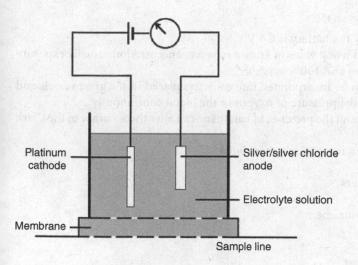

Platinum cathode

Silver/silver chloride anode

Electrolyte solution

Membrane

Sample line

1. What is this and what does it measure?
2. What is the electrolyte solution?
3. What reaction occurs at the anode?
4. What reaction occurs at the cathode?
5. What is the voltage across the cell?
6. How is this device calibrated?
7. Can this be used *in vivo*?
8. What can affect the accuracy of this device?
9. What other methods of oxygen measurement do you know?

Answers

1. This is a polarographic electrode, or Clark electrode, and it is used for measuring the partial pressure of oxygen in either liquid or gas samples.
2. The electrolyte solution is potassium chloride (some use sodium chloride).
3. Reaction at the anode:

$$Ag + Cl^- \rightarrow AgCl + e^-$$

4. Reaction at the cathode:

$$O_2 + 4e^- \rightarrow 2H_2O + 4OH^-$$

5. The voltage produced by the battery is 0.6 V.
6. Calibration is performed using gases of known oxygen concentration, usually exposure to room air (21% oxygen) and 100% oxygen.
7. Yes. Clark electrodes can be incorporated into catheters placed in the great vessels and used to measure the partial pressure of oxygen in the blood continuously.
8. Changes in temperature and the presence of halothane can alter the accuracy of the Clark electrode.
9. Other methods of oxygen measurements include:
   - Fuel cell
   - Paramagnetic analyzers
   - Mass spectrometry
   - Transcutaneous measurement

11 Oxygen Measurement 2

Questions

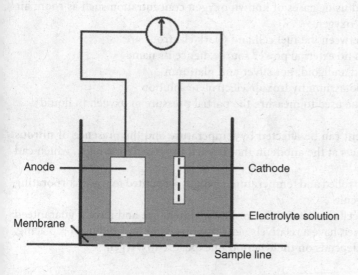

1. What is this and what does it measure?
2. What are the cathode and anode made from?
3. What is the electrolyte solution?
4. What is the reaction at the anode?
5. How is this device calibrated?
6. What are the differences between this and the Clark electrode?
7. What can affect the accuracy of this device?
8. How can the temperature of the cell be controlled?
9. What are the main advantages of this method of oxygen measurement?

Answers

1. This is a fuel cell and it is used for measuring the partial pressure of oxygen in gas samples.
2. The fuel cell has a gold mesh cathode and a lead anode.
3. The electrolyte solution is potassium hydroxide.
4. The reaction at the anode is:

$$Pb + 2OH^- \rightarrow PbO + H_2O + 2e^-$$

5. The fuel cell is calibrated using gases of known oxygen concentration such as room air (21% oxygen) and 100% oxygen.
6. The major differences between the fuel cell and Clark electrode are:
   - The fuel cell requires no external power source, hence its name
   - The fuel cell uses lead and gold, not silver and platinum
   - The fuel cell uses a potassium hydroxide electrolyte solution
   - The fuel cell cannot be used to measure the partial pressure of oxygen in liquid samples
7. Accuracy in measurement can be affected by temperature and the presence of nitrous oxide. Nitrous oxide reacts at the anode in the fuel cell to produce nitrogen, which can damage the cell.
8. Temperature can be controlled and temperature changes accounted for by incorporating a thermistor into the circuit.
9. The advantages of fuel cells are that they are low maintenance and have a guaranteed lifespan. They do, however, have a relatively slow response time and will need replacing, as their life expectancy depends on their period of exposure to oxygen.

Discussion

In the OSCE, you may get a question on oxygen measurement asking you to identify and describe a fuel cell, Clark electrode or paramagnetic analyzer. The previous two questions cover most things you will need to know about the fuel cell and Clark electrode. Be sure you know the various components of each device and the major differences between them.

The fuel cell and Clark electrode both work on a similar principle – the flow of electrons within each circuit depends on the uptake of oxygen and, in turn, depends on the partial pressure of oxygen. The greater the partial pressure, the greater the flow of current and the higher the reading given.

12 Pulmonary Artery Catheter

Pulmonary artery flotation catheters were first introduced in the 1970s by Jeremy Swan and William Ganz; hence the name Swan–Ganz catheter. Although other less invasive monitors are available, it remains the "gold standard" for cardiac ouput monitoring.

You are expected to know about Swan–Ganz catheters and could be presented with one to talk about. Knowing how to perform pulmonary artery catheterization and the route the catheter takes will help you when it comes to drawing and identifying the pulmonary artery catheter trace.

Questions

1. What is represented on this graph?

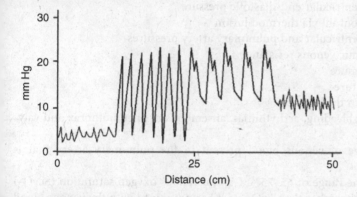

2. Describe the four stages shown.
3. Give three uses of a pulmonary artery catheter.
4. What information can you obtain from a pulmonary artery catheter?
5. How much air is in the balloon at the tip?
6. Give four complications that can arise as a result of catheter insertion.
7. What is mixed venous oxygen saturation (SvO_2) and what is the normal value?
8. In what circumstances would you get a low SvO_2?
9. What is normal pulmonary artery pressure and what values would indicate pulmonary hypertension?
10. Give three causes of pulmonary hypertension.

Answers

1. This is the trace produced by a pulmonary artery catheter as it passes through the right side of the heart and into the pulmonary vasculature.
2. *Stage 1* – The catheter passes through the right atrium; the wave form given is similar to that of the central venous pressure; pressures are 0–5 mmHg.
   Stage 2 – It passes into and through the right ventricle; the pressure wave should read between 0–5 mmHg diastolic and 20–25 mmHg systolic.
   Stage 3 – The catheter migrates into the pulmonary artery where diastolic pressures are higher at 5–12 mmHg and systolic pressure remains around 20–25 mmHg.
   Stage 4 – The balloon tip becomes wedged in one of the smaller branches of the pulmonary artery; this gives the pulmonary capillary wedge pressure (PCWP); the normal range is 6–12 mmHg.
3. Pulmonary artery catheters can be used for investigating cardiac shunts, measuring cardiac output, assessing fluid requirements in the critically ill, managing postoperative cardiac patients, assessing pulmonary hypertension and as a route for cardiac pacing.
4. Information obtained from a pulmonary artery catheter includes:
   - SvO_2
   - Estimation of left ventricular end-diastolic pressure
   - Measuring cardiac output via thermodilution
   - Right atrial, right ventricular and pulmonary artery pressures
   - Derivation of systemic venous resistance
   - Central venous pressure
   - Core body temperature
5. There is 1.5 mL of air in the balloon.
6. Complications include bleeding, arrhythmias, air embolism, pneumothorax and valvular damage.
7. SvO_2 is the percentage of venous blood present in the pulmonary artery that is oxygenated.
   Normal values lie in the range of 65–75%. Central venous oxygen saturation ($ScvO_2$) usually measures slightly higher than SvO_2, as it has not mixed with the venous blood from the coronary sinus.
8. Low SvO_2 states may be seen with:
   - Low cardiac output
   - Increasing oxygen consumption
   - Reduced arterial oxygen content; that is low hemoglobin, low arterial oxygen saturation
9. Mean pulmonary artery pressure is normally 10–15 mmHg.
   Pulmonary hypertension is defined as mean pulmonary pressure > 25 mmHg at rest or > 30 mmHg on exercise.
10. Causes of pulmonary hypertension include:
    - Chronic obstructive pulmonary disease (COPD) and interstitial lung disease
    - Recurrent pulmonary emboli
    - Left ventricular failure

Discussion

Swan–Ganz catheters are typically 70 cm long, marked every 10 cm and have a flotation balloon at the tip. They are inserted into the internal jugular or subclavian vein (using an introducer) under full sterile technique. The catheter is advanced into the right atrium where, once the pressure wave is seen, the balloon is inflated. It is then floated through the right ventricle into the pulmonary artery where it is wedged in one of the smaller arterial vessels to give the PCWP. This usually occurs at 45–55 cm but is obviously patient-dependent. The PCWP is a surrogate for left atrial filling pressure and thus representative of left ventricular end-diastolic pressure (assuming no gradient across the mitral valve or across the pulmonary capillaries. The normal range is 6–12 mmHg and is measured at the end of expiration.

A thermistor distal to the tip allows cardiac output monitoring by thermodilution methods, and fiber-optic bundles also permit continuous oximetry. True mixed venous oxygen saturations can be sampled and there is a lumen that can be used as a route for cardiac pacing.

Complications arising from insertion are similar to those of central line insertion and include bleeding, line infection, arrhythmias, air embolism, balloon rupture, pulmonary infarction and knotting of the catheter, causing valvular damage and vessel wall rupture.

Normal ranges for pulmonary artery pressure are:

Systolic	15–30 mmHg
Diastolic	0–8 mmHg
Mean	10–15 mmHg

The World Health Organization classified pulmonary hypertension into five groups:
1. Pulmonary arterial hypertension – familial, idiopathic, collagen vascular disease
2. Pulmonary hypertension associated with left heart failure – atrial, ventricular and valvular disease
3. Pulmonary hypertension associated with lung disease – COPD, interstitial lung disease, chronic hypoxemia
4. Pulmonary hypertension associated with thrombotic or embolic disease
5. Miscellaneous

13 Nerve Stimulators

There are two main types of nerve stimulator used in anesthetic practice: the *peripheral* nerve stimulator; and the *percutaneous* nerve stimulator, which is used when performing regional nerve blocks. However simple it may sound, be clear as to the differences between the two and make sure you are discussing the right type of nerve stimulator when answering the examiner's questions.

Questions

1. When would you use a *peripheral* nerve stimulator?
2. When assessing depth of neuromuscular block, where would you place the electrodes and which nerves are you stimulating?
3. What are the desired characteristics of the electrical pulse used for peripheral nerve stimulation?
4. What is train of four?
5. How is it used to assess depth of neuromuscular block?
6. Regarding the train of four, at what percentage of receptor blockade would you lose the fourth (T4) and second (T2) twitches?
7. Using the train of four, when would you consider reversal of neuromuscular blockade?
8. Describe double-burst stimulation.
9. Draw the train-of-four patterns for residual neuromuscular blockade.
10. What is meant by a supramaximal stimulus?
11. What is post-tetanic count and when is it used?
12. Other than visual assessment using the peripheral nerve stimulator, give two other methods of formally quantifying the depth of neuromuscular blockade.

Answers

1. Peripheral nerve stimulators are used during anesthesia following administration of muscle relaxants. They can be used to assess the depth of block and suitability for reversal, and guide subsequent doses of neuromuscular blocking agents.

2. Sites commonly used for nerve stimulators are:
   - *Ulnar nerve* – electrodes placed over the ulnar border of the forearm, negative electrode most distal. Produces adduction of the thumb
   - *Facial nerve* – one electrode placed in front of the tragus and the other just superior to it. Tends to be less accurate as it commonly results in direct muscle contraction and facial muscles are reportedly less sensitive to neuromuscular blockade
   - *Common peroneal nerve* – electrodes placed over the lateral aspect of the fibula neck, resulting in dorsiflexion of the foot

3. Ideally, the electrical pulse produced should be of uniform current amplitude (10–50 mA) with a square wave form and of a duration around 0.2 ms.

4. Train of four is a particular pattern of stimulation, consisting of four identical stimuli given at a frequency of 2 Hz (four pulses, 0.5 s apart).

5. In the presence of non-depolarizing muscle relaxants, the height or magnitude of the twitches varies depending on the degree of neuromuscular block present.
   Muscle twitch height will diminish from the first to the fourth in the presence of neuromuscular blockade. With a profound block you may only see the first twitch. The height of the fourth twitch (T4) compared to the first twitch (T1) gives a T4:T1 ratio, which is indicative of the depth of neuromuscular block.

6. T4, the fourth twitch, is lost at 75–80% acetylcholine receptor occupancy. T2, the second twitch, is lost at 85–90% acetylcholine receptor occupancy.

7. Reversal with neostigmine or edrophonium can be considered when there are three to four detectable twitches on train of four or the T4:T1 ratio is greater than 0.7. Sugammadex can be used for more intense blocks.

8. Double-burst stimulation consists of two distinct clusters of stimulation at 50 Hz. Each burst is composed of three pulses at 20-ms intervals and each burst is separated by 0.75 s.

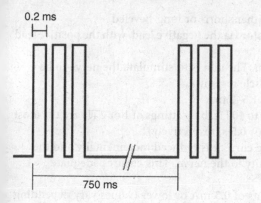

9.

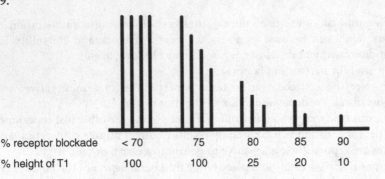

% receptor blockade	< 70	75	80	85	90
% height of T1	100	100	25	20	10

10. A supramaximal stimulus is an electrical stimulus with magnitude significantly above that required to depolarize all nerve or muscle fibers in a given region.
11. Post-tetanic count is used in circumstances of profound neuromuscular block when train of four or double-burst stimulation is not useful.

    The anesthesiologist produces an initial phase of tetany within the muscle, this tetanic burst is given at 50 Hz for 5 s. Following tetany, electrical stimuli are administered at 1 Hz (i.e. one per second), and the number of resultant twitches recorded.

    A post-tetanic count of less than 5 indicates deep neuromuscular block, whereas a count of more than 15 indicates that reversal of blockade may be possible.
12. Methods such as mechanomyography and acceleromyography may be used although these methods are time-consuming and results can be inconsistent.

Discussion

Peripheral nerve stimulators offer a simple and, if used correctly, a reliable means of assessing the depth of neuromuscular blockade. Their use is indicated during any anesthetic where muscle relaxation is required.

You may also be asked about *percutaneous* nerve stimulators. The salient points of these are:

- They use insulated stimulating needles, either short- or long-beveled
- The needle is attached to the nerve stimulator via the negative lead, with the positive lead grounded via the patient
- The needle is introduced through the skin. The aim is to stimulate the nerve to be blocked by producing an appropriate muscle response
- They use lower currents, starting around 1.5–2 mA
- The frequency of impulse can vary from 1 to 10 Hz, but settings of 1 or 2 Hz are the most common (producing an impulse every 1 or 0.5 s, respectively)
- Once muscle contraction is identified, the current is reduced incrementally and the needle advanced carefully to gain proximity to the nerve. This ensures adequate blockade once local anesthetic is injected
- Note that muscle contraction with currents of 0.3 mA or lower (values vary depending on the literature) can indicate that the needle is lying within the nerve itself. The needle should be withdrawn and no local anesthetic infiltrated

14 Pulse Oximetry

The commercialization of pulse oximetry in the 1980s was an incredible step forward for medicine as a whole. None of us today would dream of giving an anesthetic without a pulse oximeter, and for this reason it is, like capnography, a potential examination question.

Questions
1. What two physical principles is pulse oximetry based on?
2. Look at the following diagram. Identify the traces shown.

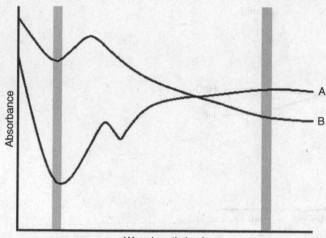

3. What wavelengths of light are used?
4. What is the isosbestic point?
5. What information can be gained from a pulse oximetry trace?
6. What factors affect the accuracy of pulse oximetry?
7. Are there any limitations to the use of pulse oximetry?
8. What factors affect oxygen delivery to body tissue?
9. Define hypoxia.
10. Give three causes of hypoxemic hypoxia.

Answers

1. Pulse oximetry is based on Beer's law and Lambert's law.
   - *Beer's law* – the amount of light absorbed when passing through a medium is proportional to the concentration of the medium
   - *Lambert's law* – the amount of light absorbed when passing through a medium is proportional to the thickness of the medium
2. A: Oxygenated hemoglobin (HbO_2)
   B: Deoxygenated hemoglobin (Hb)
3. The wavelengths used are those of red and infrared light; they are 660 nm and 940 nm, respectively.

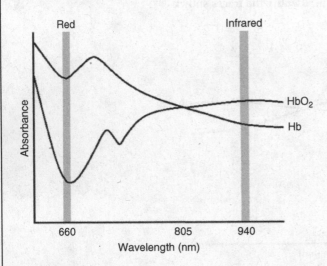

4. The isosbestic point is the wavelength at which deoxyhemoglobin and oxyhemoglobin have the same absorptive capacity. In this case it occurs at 805 nm.
5. From the pulse oximetry trace you can obtain information about:
   - Arterial oxygen saturation (SpO_2)
   - Heart rate
   - Cardiac output
6. Excessive amounts of ambient light and low output states will cause inaccuracy. Malpositioning of the probe and venous congestion can result in under-reading. Methemoglobin, carboxyhemoglobin and the use of methylene blue in surgery will all affect the accuracy of pulse oximetry.
7. Limitations to use include:
   - Only accurate in the SpO_2 range of 70–100%
   - There is a time lag of around 30–60 s depending on the position of the probe; changes in saturation, therefore, are not picked up immediately
   - Burns have been reported, so it is recommended probes are moved every few hours in long-term use
   - Can be inaccurate in the presence of arrhythmias and hypotension
   - It relies on delicate electrical components and may malfunction if damaged

8. Factors affecting oxygen delivery are cardiac output, hemoglobin concentration, arterial oxygen saturation of hemoglobin and the arterial partial pressure of oxygen.
9. Hypoxia refers to a state in which body tissue as a whole has an inadequate supply of oxygen. Hypoxia can be classified as ischemic, cytotoxic, hypoxemic and anemic.
10. Hypoxemic hypoxia occurs in:
   - Shunt
   - V/Q mismatch
   - Hypoventilation
   - Reduced partial pressure of inspired oxygen

Discussion

Knowledge of pulse oximetry is a vital piece of the examination curriculum. You must know how it works, what it measures and what its uses and limitations are.

It may come up as an OSCE station and may well be linked with the oxyhemoglobin dissociation curve. Remember:
- The P_{50} is the partial pressure of oxygen (PO_2) at which blood is 50% saturated
- The P_{50} is commonly quoted as 27 mmHg
- Venous blood has a PO_2 of 40 mmHg when about 75% saturated
- Arterial blood has a PO_2 of 100 mmHg when about 98% saturated

Plotting these values on a labelled axis and drawing an accurate hemoglobin dissociation curve will score well.

Factors shifting the curve to the *left*: hypothermia, hypocarbia, alkalosis and reduced levels of 2,3-diphosphoglycerate (2,3-DPG).

Factors shifting the curve to the *right*: hyperthermia, hypercarbia, acidosis and raised levels of 2,3-DPG.

15 Rotameters

For many years, rotameters have been an integral part of the anesthetic machine, forming the rotameter block, where gas flows are measured and altered by the anesthesiologist. Some of the modern anesthetic machines employ electronic flow-meters, and rotameters are no longer part of the display panel.

It is a topic that may be examined as it neatly brings together physics and clinical measurement.

Questions

1. What is this and what does it measure?

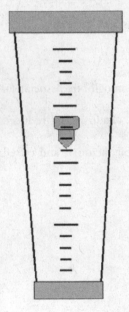

2. What are the working principles behind this flow-meter?
3. How does gas flow vary from the bottom to the top of the rotameter?
4. What equation exists for flow at the top of the rotameter?
5. What properties does the bobbin possess and at what level do you read the bobbin?
6. Why are rotameters gas-specific?
7. What are the advantages of rotameters?
8. Do they have any limitations?
9. How is gas flow through the rotameter regulated?
10. What are the safety features of the rotameter block?

Answers

1. This is a rotameter and it measures the flow rate of a gas or liquid.
2. Rotameters are variable-orifice, constant-pressure, flow-meters. The tapered tube means that the orifice around the bobbin varies, depending on gas flow. At high gas flows the bobbin is further from the tube sides than at low gas flow. The pressure across the bobbin remains constant as it balances the forces of gravity and flow.
3. Gas flow at the bottom of the rotameter behaves as in a tube and, therefore, is laminar. As you go further up the rotameter, gas flows as it would through an orifice and becomes turbulent.
4. Flow at the top is turbulent; the equation for the Reynolds number (Re) is:

    $$Re = \frac{density \times velocity \times diameter}{viscosity}$$

    A Reynolds number greater than 2,000 indicates that flow is likely to be turbulent.
5. The bobbins are made of light metals, specific to a given gas, and have slits in them to help rotation and reduce sticking. Readings are taken from the upper surface of the bobbin. Plastic balls can be used but may be less accurate.
6. Flow at the top of the tube is turbulent and, therefore, density-dependent. Flow at the bottom of the tube is laminar and viscosity-dependent. As gases have different densities and viscosities, flow-meters have to be calibrated for a specific gas.
7. Advantages of rotameters:
    *   Cheap and easy to construct
    *   Simple and reliable
    *   They depend on gas flow and not a power supply
    *   They have no electronic display or component to malfunction
8. Limitations of rotameters:
    *   They must be kept vertical to function accurately
    *   They are calibrated only for a specific gas
    *   Bobbins can stick due to build-up of electrical charge or dirt
    *   They can crack, producing inaccurate readings
    *   Backpressure from the circuit can also affect flow measurements
9. Gas flow is controlled by a needle valve at the base of the flow-meter.
10. The built-in safety features include:
    *   Color-coded knobs for different gases
    *   Different shaped knobs for gases, with oxygen being the largest
    *   Conducting strips to reduce build-up of static charge
    *   Nitrous oxide and oxygen rotameters are linked to prevent delivery of a hypoxic gas mixture ("hypoxic guard")
    *   Oxygen should be arranged so that it enters downstream of other gases, thus preventing the delivery of a hypoxic gas mixture

Discussion

Rotameters are variable-orifice, constant-pressure, flow-meters. They consist of a tapered glass tube, a needle valve to control gas flow, a bobbin and a conducting strip. The tapered tube has markings on its walls, giving measurements of low gas flows at the bottom and high gas flows at the top. Readings are taken from the top of a metal alloy bobbin or from the middle of a plastic ball bobbin.

In order to obtain accurate readings, the flow-meter must be kept vertical and calibrated for a specific gas. Bobbins can stick and so they contain slits in them to aid rotation, and some possess a conducting strip to carry away static charge to prevent sticking.

Flow-meters have been quoted as being accurate within 2.5% of true flow value.

There is a mixture of both laminar and turbulent flow in a rotameter:

- Laminar flow exists at low flows – the Hagen–Poiseuille equation
- Turbulent flow exists at high flows – dictated by Reynolds number

Thus, at the bottom of the tube flow depends on the viscosity, at the top of the tube flow depends on density. Hence, all rotameters are calibrated using a specific gas owing to variations in viscosity and density.

You may well be asked about the problems surrounding positioning of gases on a rotameter block. It is enough to say that oxygen should enter downstream of the other gases to prevent delivery of a hypoxic gas mixture in the event that one of the other flow-meters develops a fault.

16 Temperature

Much like humidity, temperature is a very clinically important topic. It houses a variety of important terms and definitions that you must learn as well as a number of measuring devices that you could be asked to describe and explain.

As anesthesiologists, we are responsible for maintaining and monitoring the patient's temperature during surgical procedures. There are different routes by which temperature can be measured and various ways of warming patients; this has been examined in the past!

Questions

1. What is this and what does it measure?

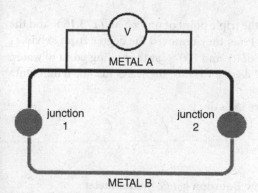

2. What is the principle on which it is based?
3. What different metals are commonly used?
4. What is the triple point of water?
5. What is core temperature?
6. Describe two different temperature scales.
7. What other methods do you know for measuring temperature?
8. Draw graphs of resistance against temperature for:
   - A thermistor
   - A resistance thermometer
9. Give some disadvantages of mercury thermometers.
10. Why would alcohol be used instead of mercury in a thermometer?
11. Give the major routes of heat loss from the human body.

Answers

1. This is a thermocouple. It measures temperature.
2. Thermocouples are based on the Seebeck effect. This dictates that the voltage produced at a junction of two dissimilar metals is dependent on temperature. If you have one junction kept at a constant temperature (reference junction) and another junction measuring atmospheric temperature, the difference in voltage between the two will be proportional to the difference in temperature.
3. The metals commonly used are nickel–constantan and platinum–rhodium. Constantan is an alloy of nickel (45%) and copper (55%).
4. The triple point of water is the temperature at which the three phases of water (gas, liquid and solid) exist in thermodynamic equilibrium. It is given as 0.01 °C (273.16 K).
5. Core body temperature refers to the temperature of the central organs such as the brain, abdominal and thoracic contents and the proximal deep tissues of the limbs, which is maintained by homeostatic mechanisms. Core body temperature normally ranges from 36.5 °C to 37.5 °C. Variation occurs naturally as a result of our circadian rhythm.
6. Kelvin (K) and Celsius (°C) are two types of temperature scale. There is also the Fahrenheit scale.
   Kelvin – absolute zero is given as 0 K with the triple point of water being 273.16 K and the boiling point of water being 373.16 K. In 1968, they removed the degree from kelvin.
   Celsius – 0 °C is given as the melting point of ice and 100 °C as the boiling point of water. A change of one kelvin is the same as one degree Celsius; the scales just have different starting points.
7. Other methods for measuring temperature include:
   - Thermistor
   - Wire resistor
   - Bimetallic strip
   - Liquid thermometer
   - Gas expansion thermometer such as the Bourdon gauge thermometer
   - Infrared thermometer
   - Thermopile – a series of thermocouples

8.

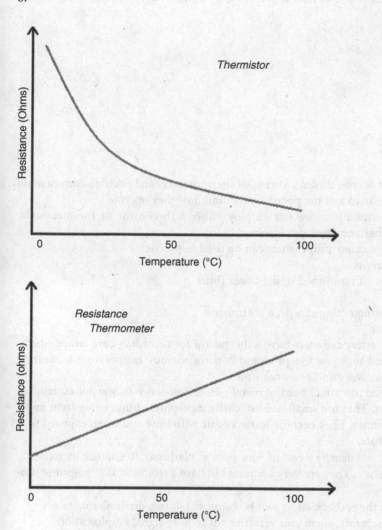

9. They are fragile and difficult to insert into certain body regions, there is the risk of spilling mercury as well as breaking the glass and they take around two minutes to take an accurate reading.

10. Ethanol freezes at −114 °C and boils at 78.4 °C.
    Mercury freezes at −39 °C and boils at 356.7 °C.
    Alcohol thermometers, therefore, are useful at lower temperatures. They are also cheaper than mercury thermometers, and, if they break, are not considered a toxic or hazardous material.

11. There are four major routes of heat loss from the human body:

Respiration	10%
Evaporation	20%
Convection	30%
Radiation	40%

Discussion

In the examination, you may be shown a variety of thermometers and asked to comment on where and how they are used and the principles behind how they operate.

The majority of thermometers we use employ either a thermistor or thermocouple. Tympanic membrane thermometers use infrared.

Various sites for measuring temperature can be used in practice:

- Mouth and nasopharynx
- Esophagus – accurate if positioned in the lower third
- Rectum and axilla
- Bladder – urinary catheter tipped with a thermistor
- Tympanic membrane
- Blood – pulmonary artery catheters have a thermistor for recording core temperature

You will be expected to know the pros and cons of various temperature-measuring techniques, including accuracy and response times.

Thermistor – composed of a small bead of metal oxide. Resistance falls exponentially as temperature increases. They are small, robust, easily incorporated into equipment and have rapid response times. They become less accurate with time and when exposed to extremes of temperature.

Resistance thermometer – usually a coil of wire such as platinum. Resistance increases linearly with temperature. They are very accurate but have a relatively slow response time and are fragile.

Thermocouple – uses the Seebeck effect and is composed of two dissimilar metals. Thermocouples are accurate, small and versatile but require signal amplification.

Bimetallic strip – composed of two metals in a coil or strip attached to a pointer. As the temperature rises or falls the metals expand and contract to move the pointer over a given scale. They are robust, cheap and provide continuous measurement but are relatively inaccurate.

Infrared thermometers – these detect infrared radiation emitted at the tympanic membrane as heat is lost via the ear canal. They have quick response times and are accurate. However, they do run the risk of perforating the ear drum.

Further Reading List

Allman KG, Wilson IH. *Oxford Handbook of Anaesthesia*, 2nd edn. Oxford University Press, 2006.

Al-Shaikh B. *Essentials of Anaesthetic Equipment*. Churchill Livingstone, 1995.

Cross M, Plunkett E. *Physics, Pharmacology and Physiology for Anaesthetists*. Cambridge University Press, 2008.

Davis PD, Kenny GNC. *Basic Physics and Measurement in Anaesthesia*. Butterworth Heineman, 2003.

Deakin C. *Clinical Notes for the FRCA*. Churchill Livingstone, 2011.

Hampton JR. *The ECG Made Easy*, 5th edn. Churchill Livingstone, 1998.

Marik PE, Baram M, Vahid B. Does central venous pressure predict fluid responsiveness? A systematic review of the literature and the tale of seven mares. *Chest*, 2008, **134**: 172–8.

McFadyen G. *Update in Anaesthesia – Respiratory Gas Analysis*. Available from: www.anaesthesiologists.org.

Shippy CR, Appel PL, Shoemaker WC. Reliability of clinical monitoring to assess blood volume in critically ill patients. *Crit Care Med*, 1984, **12**: 107–112.

Smith T, Pinnock C, Lin T. *Fundamentals of Anaesthesia*, 3rd edn. Cambridge University Press, 2002.

West JB. *Respiratory Physiology: The Essentials*, 7th edn. Lippincott Williams and Wilkins, 2005.

Yentis S, Hirsch N, Smith G. *Anaesthesia and Intensive Care A–Z*. Churchill Livingstone, 2009.

Index

Printed in the United States
by Baker & Taylor Publisher Services